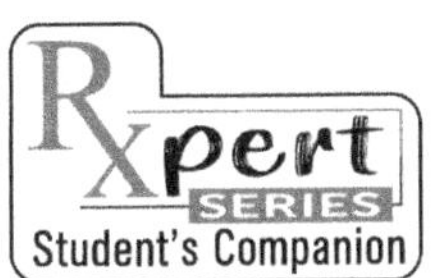

Pharmaceutical Organic Chemistry-I

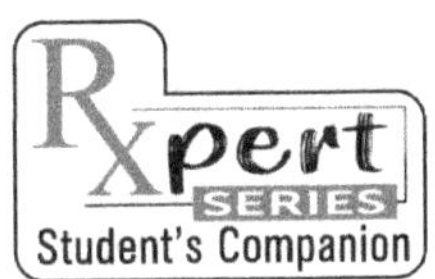

Pharmaceutical Organic Chemistry-I

Dr. Pooja A Chawla

PhD, M Pharm

Professor and Head
Department of Pharmaceutical Chemistry and Analysis
ISF College of Pharmacy, Moga,142001, Punjab

Ms. Simranpreet Kaur Wahan

MSc

Assistant Professor
ISF College of Pharmacy, Moga

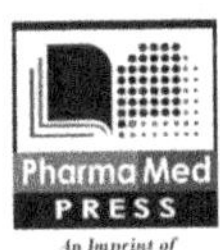

PharmaMed Press

An imprint of BSP Books Pvt. Ltd

4-4-309/316, Giriraj Lane,
Sultan Bazar, Hyderabad - 500 095.

Pharmaceutical Organic Chemistry-I

by **Dr. Pooja A. Chawla and Simranpreet Kaur Wahan**

© 2023, *by Publisher*

Disclaimer: The authors and the publishers have taken due care to provide the authentic, reliable and up to date information related to the subject. However, neither the authors nor the publisher shall be responsible for any liability for any damage caused as a result of use of this book. The respective user must check the accuracy from other sources too.

Published by:

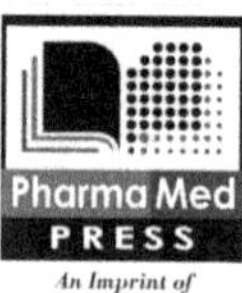

PharmaMed Press

An imprint of BSP Books Pvt. Ltd.
4-4-309/316, Giriraj Lane, Sultan Bazar, Hyderabad - 500 095.
Phone: 040-23445688; Fax: 91+40-23445611
e-mail: info@pharmamedpress.com
www.pharmamedpress.com/pharmamedpress.net

ISBN: 978-93-95039-19-2 (Hardback)

Preface

The concepts of organic chemistry are vast and demand a thorough reading for understanding. As a part of curriculum at diploma/undergraduate/postgraduate level, a pharmacy student has to read Pharmaceutical Organic Chemistry. The evolution of this book is a culmination of efforts by the authors to make the concepts clear in an easy to understand language. The primary objective of this book is to make the students aware about the key curriculum points in B Pharmacy Second Semester subject of Pharmaceutical Organic Chemistry-I. The book enables the reader to write the structure, name and types of isomerism, reactions, and names of reactions and orientation of reactions related to organic compounds. It also equips the reader to account for reactivity and stability of compounds and to identify and confirm the identity of organic compounds. The text has been enriched with a detailed write up on various mechanisms where required. It prepares the readers for the various competitive examinations and end semester examination.

While every effort has been made to keep errors at bay, few errors might have still crept in. Your feedback is solicited and shall be highly appreciated.

- Authors

Contents

Unit – 1

Classification, Nomenclature and Isomerism

Unit – 2

Alkanes, Alkanes and Conjugated Dienes

Unit – 3

Alkyl Halides and Alcohols

Unit – 4

Carbonyl Compounds

Unit – 5

Carboxylic Acids and Amines

Unit - 1

Classification, Nomenclature and Isomerism

- Organic chemistry is the branch of chemistry which deals with carbon containing compounds.
- Carbon atoms show highest catenation property. Carbon atoms form chains and rings of various sizes and branching.
- The various compounds of different sizes and structures corresponds to different physical and chemical properties.
- Organic chemistry holds much importance in technological world. The various dyes, pharmaceuticals, paper, paints, pesticides, insecticides, petroleum-based products, rubber tyres etc. all come under organic chemistry.
- Organic chemistry is a hugely important field in technology: it's the chemistry of dyes and pharmaceuticals, paper and ink, paints and plastics, gasoline; it's the chemistry of the food we eat and the clothes we wear.
- Organic chemistry is critical in biology and medicine. Apart from water, biological creatures are mostly composed of organic compounds; the molecules of "molecular biology" are organic compounds.
- Organic chemistry also includes carbon compounds such as cholesterol and polyunsaturated fats, growth hormones and steroids, insecticides, and many others. In addition to carbon and hydrogen, organic molecules include a vast variety of medicinal compounds that contain other heteroatoms such as O, N, S, and so on in their chemical structures.
- These compounds have wide-ranging therapeutic effect such as anti-malarial, anti-inflammatory, anti-cancer, anti-viral, anti-fungal, and so on.

Nomenclature of Organic Compounds

Two general ways of naming organic compounds have been in practice:

1. Trivial System

In which the compounds are named after the source from which they are obtained or from their characteristic property.

For example:

$HCOOH$ -Formic acid (red ants)

CH_3COOH-Acetic acid (acetum-vinegar)

2. IUPAC system: (International Union of Pure and Applied Chemistry)

It is most scientific and universally accepted used for nomenclature of organic compounds. Certain set of rules are to be followed for assigning IUPAC names of various organic compounds. The names assigned by following IUPAC rules are termed as systematic names. The name of the compound obtained by adding suffix and prefix to the name of the unbranched hydrocarbons. The base of the name indicates the length of the chain or ring i.e., the number of carbons atoms present in the parent compound. The suffix is added to parent name which indicates the type of functional group present in the parent chain. Prefix is used to indicate the substituent present in the organic compound.

The IUPAC name of the compound consists of:

- Prefix
- Word root
- Primary suffix
- Secondary suffix

ubstituent group	Prefix
-F	Fluoro
-Cl	Chloro
-Br	Bromo
-I	Iodo
$-NO_2$	Nitro
$-CH_3$	Methyl
$-C_2H_5$	Ethyl
$-C_3H_7$	Propyl

Word Root

Number of Carbons	Name
1	meth
2	eth
3	prop
4	but
5	pent
6	hex
7	hept
8	oct
9	non
10	dec
11	undec
12	dodec

It indicates the number of carbon atoms in the longest possible chain.

Primary Suffix:

Primary suffix indicates the type of carbon-carbon bond in the organic compound.

$$\text{ane: } \quad — \quad \text{bond}$$
$$\text{ene: } \quad = \quad \text{bond}$$
$$\text{yne: } \quad \equiv \quad \text{bond}$$

Secondary suffix: It represents the functional group if present in an organic molecule and is attached to the primary suffix while writing the IUPAC name. Priorities of Substituents and Functional Groups LISTED HERE FROM HIGHEST TO LOWEST PRIORITY. Many organic compounds contain more than one functional group. In those cases the functional group of highest priority is termed as suffix and in known as principal group. The functional group of lowest priority is known as junior group is added as prefix. The following order of priority is used for selecting the principal and functional group:

Carboxylic acids>sulphonic acids>acid anhydrides>esters>acid halides>amides>nitriles>aldehydes>ketones>alcohols>amines>ethers

Functional group	Prefix name	Suffix name
Carboxylic acid	carboxy	-oic acid
Ester	Alkoxycarbonyl	-oate
Amide	Amido	-amide
Nitrile	Nitrile	cyano
Aldehyde	Formyl	-al
Ketone	Oxo	-one
Alcohol	Hydroxy	-ol
Amine	Amino	-amine
Ether	Alkoxy	-
Alkyl Halide	Halo	-

IUPAC = prefix +word root + primary suffix +secondary suffix

Writing IUPAC name of an aliphatic compound

Eg:

$$\underset{3}{CH_3}-\underset{2}{CH}-\overset{H_2}{\underset{1}{C}}-OH$$
$$\quad\quad\quad | \quad$$
$$\quad\quad\quad CH_3$$

Word root: prop

Prefix: methyl

Primary suffix: ane

Secondary suffix: ol

IUPAC name- 2-Methyl-1-propanol

Rules of Writing Iupac Names

1. Select the largest chain

Side chain is at C_3
(right)

Side chain is at C_5
(left)

2. Numbering of carbon is done from the side   in order to give least possible number to the side chain. Side chain derived from alkane is called alkyl. Alkyl group can be primary, secondary and tertiary.

    (a) The prefix n-(normal) refers to a straight chain alkyl, without any branching or cross links in the chain.

    (b) The prefix iso is used when all carbons atoms except one are present in straight continuous chain.

    (c) The prefix s- is read as secondary, indicates linking at a secondary carbon that is, one bound to two carbons.

    (d) The prefix t- is read as tertiary to indicate attachment at a tertiary carbon-that is one bound to three other carbons.

3. If more than one side is present, sum of the positions should be minimum while numbering the carbon chain

sum of positions: 5+5+7=17
(wrong)

sum of positions: 3+5+5=13
(right)

4. If two different alkyl groups are at equal positions from each other end, numbering is done from the side of the smaller alkyl group.

5. When the substituents are other than alkyl groups, numbers are assigned in the alphabetical order.

6. When a compound contains a functional group, the lowest number is assigned to the functional group and to the substituent, even if it violates the minimum sum rule.

7. For compounds with more than one functional group. Following order is followed in assigning principal and junior functional group:

Carboxylic acids>sulphonic acids>acid anhydrides>esters>acid
halides>amides>nitriles>aldehydes>ketones>alcohols>amines>ethers

In the compound given below keto group is junior (prefix) functional group whereas aldehyde is principal functional group.

Principal group

$CH_3-C-CHO$
$\quad\ \ \overset{\|}{O}$

2-keto (or oxo) propanal

Isomers

The compounds having same molecular formula but different properties due to different arrangement of atoms in the molecule are termed as isomers. There are two types of isomerism:

- **Structural Isomerism**
- **Stereo Isomerism**

Structural Isomerism: The structural isomers are those with different atomic arrangement of molecules without regard for spatial arrangement in 3-D space. Constitutional isomerism and structural isomerism are two terms for the same thing.

In other words, while they have same molecular formula they possess different structures. This type of isomerism which arises from difference in the structure of molecules, includes:

1. **Chain or Nuclear Isomerism;**
2. **Positional Isomerism**
3. **Functional Isomerism**
4. **Metamerism**
5. **Tautomerism**

Stereochemistry is the discipline of chemistry that studies "the various spatial configurations of atoms in molecules."

Stereochemistry is the methodical exposition of a specific topic of science and technology that generally necessitates a little detour into history. Stereochemistry is known as the "chemistry of space," since it deals with the spatial arrangements of atoms and groups in a molecule. Stereochemistry is known as the "chemistry of space," since it deals with the spatial arrangements of atoms and groups in a molecule.

Stereochemistry may be traced back to 1842, when the French chemist Louis Pasteur discovered that tartaric acid salts obtained from a wine production vessel had the capacity to rotate plane-polarized light, but the identical salts from various sources do not. Optical isomerism gives explanation of this phenomena.

1. Chain Isomerism

- Isomers are chain isomers, which occur when two or more compounds have the same chemical formula but vary in the carbon atom branching. It is sometimes referred to as skeletal isomerism. These isomers' constituents have a variety of branching structures.

- Typically, chain isomers differ in the degree of carbon branching.

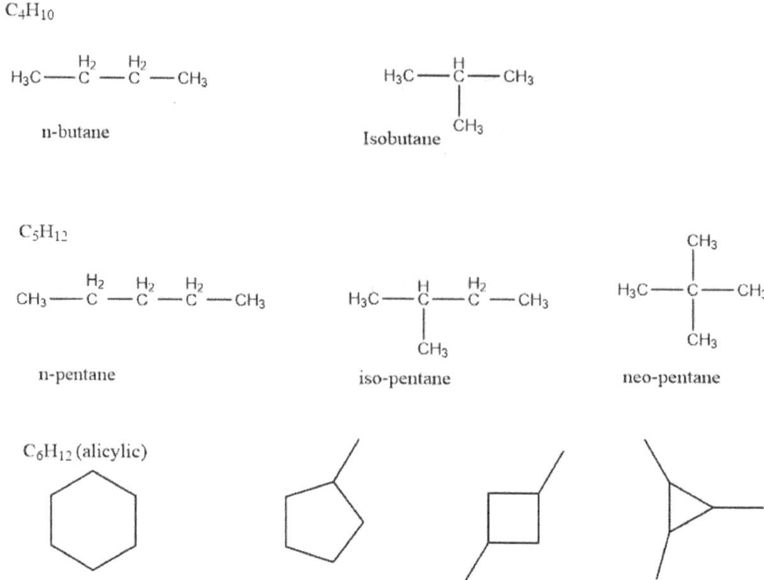

2. **Position Isomerism**

Position isomers are compounds having different location of the functional group or substituent atoms. In position isomers, the locations of the functional groups or substituent atoms vary along the chain.

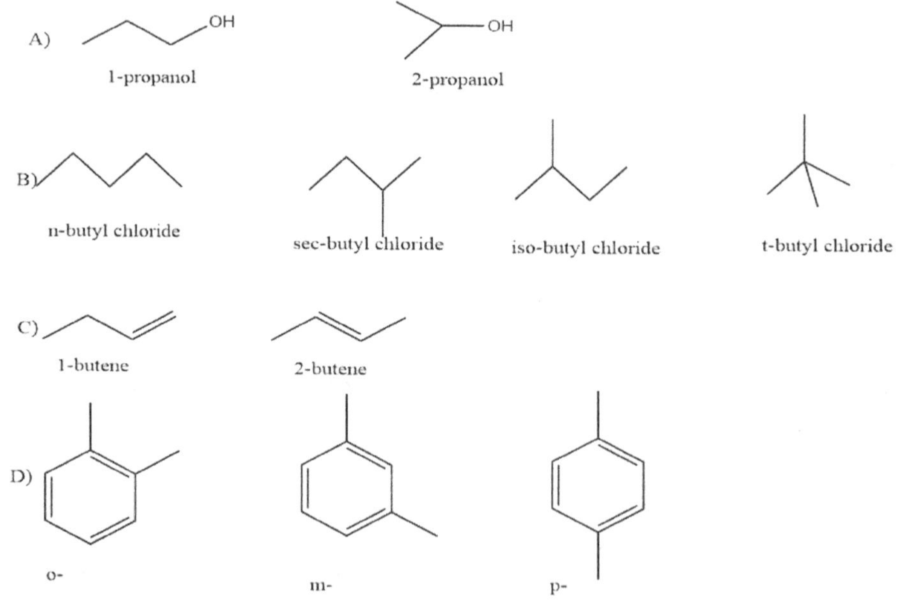

3. Functional Isomerism

Isomers are functional isomers when two or more compounds have the same chemical formula but have different functional groups present in them. It is sometimes referred to as functional group isomerism.

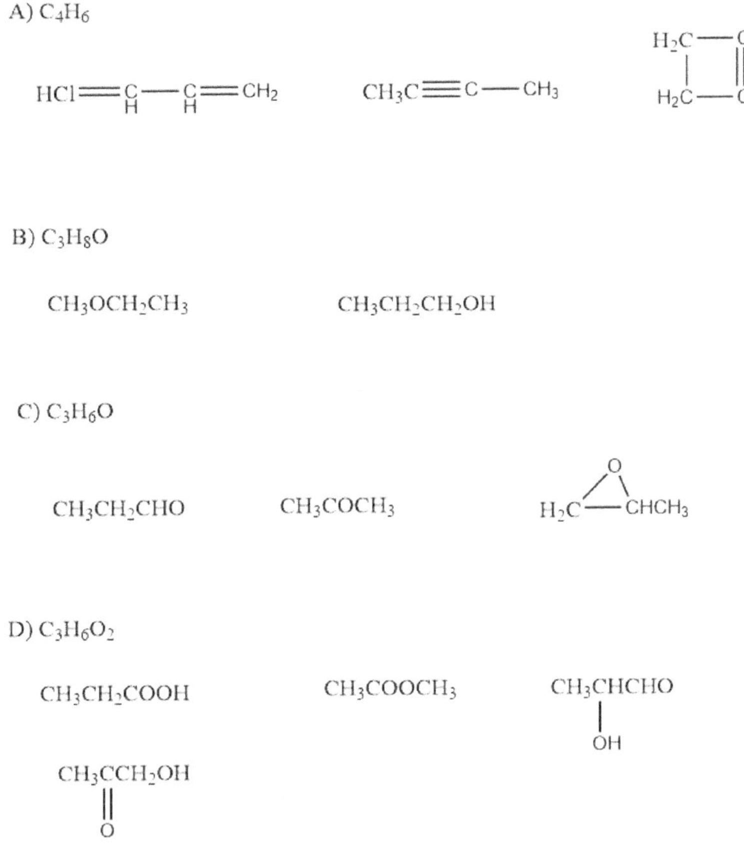

A) C_4H_6

B) C_3H_8O

$CH_3OCH_2CH_3$ $CH_3CH_2CH_2OH$

C) C_3H_6O

CH_3CH_2CHO CH_3COCH_3

D) $C_3H_6O_2$

CH_3CH_2COOH CH_3COOCH_3 CH_3CHCHO

4. Metamerism

Metamerism arises when distinct alkyl chains are present on the either side of the functional group. It is a type of isomerism that occurs only in compounds having a divalent element (sulphur or oxygen) having alkyl groups on both the sides.

A) H_3CH_2C—O—CH_2CH_3 H_3C—O—$CH_2CH_2CH_3$

Dimethyl ether   Methyl propyl ether

B) H_3CH_2C—$\overset{H}{N}$—CH_2CH_3 $H_3CH_2CH_2C$—$\overset{H}{N}$—CH_3

Diethylamine   Methylpropylamine

5. Tautomerism

Tautomers of the compound have different location of protons and electrons. Carbonyls exhibit keto-enol tautomerism due to the acidity of hydrogens. Tautomers are constitutional isomers that are rapidly interconverted. Under typical conditions, the equilibrium between tautomers is not only quick, but it frequently favours one of the isomers (acetone, for example, is 99.9% keto tautomer).

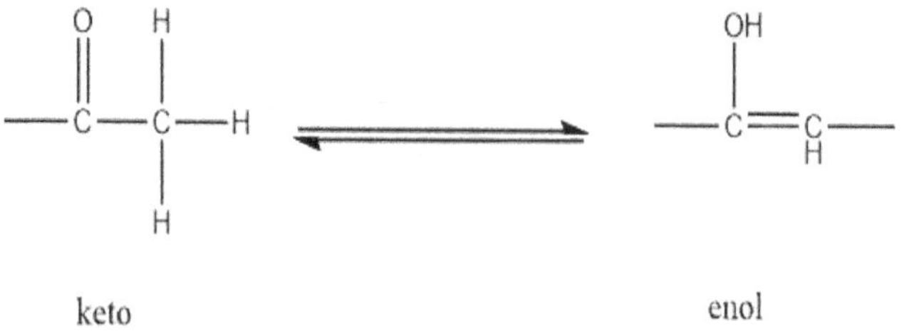

keto   enol

- The tautomers of a chemical exist in equilibrium with each other and easily exchange.
- This occurs through intramolecular transfer of proton. Keto-enol tautomerism is a prominent example. Tautomerism basically happens in the presence of a catalyst.
- Acid-catalyst: Protonation occurs first, followed by cation delocalization. The cation deprotonates at the neighbouring site.
- Deprotonation is the initial step in the production of base catalysts. Instead of cation delocalization, anion delocalization occurs, followed by protonation to a new anion location.

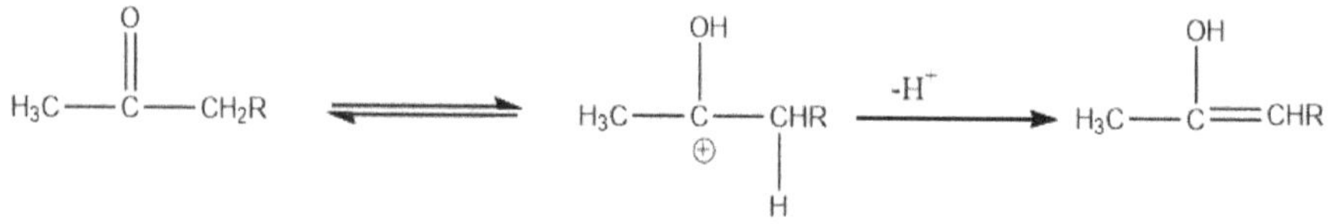

ACID CATALYSED CONVERSION

One of the most important characteristics of tautomerism is that it increases the stability of the chemical compound. In this process, a hydrogen atom is exchanged between two other atoms while creating a covalent bond to either one. Structural requirement of Tautomerism are as follows:

- ✓ Compounds comprise polar molecules and functional groups with weakly acidic groups.
- ✓ It has no influence on bond length or other characteristics.
- ✓ It often occurs in planar or non-planar molecules.

$$H_3C-\overset{\overset{\displaystyle O}{\|}}{C}-CH_2R \underset{-H_2O}{\overset{OH^-}{\rightleftharpoons}} H_3C-\overset{\overset{\displaystyle O}{\|}}{C}-\overset{\ominus}{C}HR \underset{-OH^-}{\overset{H_2O}{\longrightarrow}} H_3C-\overset{\overset{\displaystyle OH}{|}}{C}=CHR$$

keto

enolic form

enolic form

keto form

$$HO-C\equiv N \rightleftharpoons O=C=N-H$$

Cyanic acid   Isocyanic acid

$$H_3C-\overset{\overset{\displaystyle O}{\|}}{C}-\overset{H_2}{C}-\overset{\overset{\displaystyle O}{\|}}{C}-OC_2H_5 \overset{H^+ \text{ or } OH^-}{\rightleftharpoons} H_3C-\overset{\overset{\displaystyle OH}{|}}{C}=\overset{}{\underset{H}{C}}-\overset{\overset{\displaystyle O}{\|}}{C}-OC_2H_5$$

(keto form)
acetoacetic ester

(enolic form)

Tautomerism Types

Emil Erlenmeyer, a scientist, developed the rule for tautomerism in the 1880s. He was among the first to explore the keto-enol tautomerism. According to this rule, the hydroxyl group in all alcohols generates ketones or aldehydes when it is directly connected to a double-bonded carbon atom. This was attributable to the increased stability of the keto form.

There are other forms of tautomerism, but keto-enol tautomerism is the most common. One structure in this form is a ketone, while the other is an enol. By using acid or basic catalysts, both tautomeric forms can be interconverted to one other. Enolization is the process of converting a ketone to an enol.

Prototropy

It is a form of tautomerism caused by the compound's acid-base behaviour. The sole difference between these two versions is the location of a proton. This structure will use the same empirical formula and numbers of charges as the previous one.

Annular Tautomerism

An annular tautomerism occurs when a proton occupies two or more positions in a heterocyclic system. If an open structure in tautomerism is converted to a ring structure owing to proton delocalization, then such tautomers are known as ring-chain tautomers. Ring-chain tautomerism is also studied in glucose.

Valence Tautomerism

Valence tautomerism is a kind of tautomerism in which single and double bonds are continuously formed and broken in the compound without any movement of groups or atoms. It differs from the preceding form of tautomerism in that it occurs quickly.

There is a shift in geometrical structure but no change in canonical resonance structure or mesomers in this tautomerism.

MCQs

1. Give the IUPAC name of given compound

$$HC \equiv\!\!\!-\!\!\!-\!\!\!\equiv CH_2$$

   (a) Pent-1-en-4-yne   (b) Pent-4-en-1-yne

   (c) Pent-5-yne-1-ene   (d) Pent-1-yne-5-ene

2. The number of sigma and pi bond in the compound pent-3-en-1-yne

   (a) 10, 3   (b) 3, 10

   (c) 9, 4   (d) 8, 3

3. An isomer of ethanol

   (a) Methanol   (b) Diethyl ether

   (c) Dimethyl ether   (d) Acetone

4. Compounds having same molecular formula but different structures are called:

   (a) Structural isomers   (b) Molecular isomer

   (c) Optical isomers   (d) Position isomers

5. A monocarboxylic is functional isomer of

   (a) Ether   (b) Amine

   (c) Ester   (d) Alcohol

6. Which is correct for 3,4-dibromo1-pentene and 3,5-dibromo-2-pentene

   I. They have same molecular formula $C_5H_8Br_2$

   II. They are positional isomers

   III. They have same chemical properties

   (a) I and II
   (b) I and III
   (c) II and III
   (d) I, II and III

7. The isomers has:

   (a) Same chemical properties
   (b) Same molecular formula
   (c) Same structural formula
   (d) Same functional groups

8. Ethanol (C_2H_5OH) and dimethyl ether (CH_3OCH_3) are:

   (a) Functional isomer
   (b) Position isomers
   (c) Metamers
   (d) Chain isomers

9. The compound $CH_3CH_2OCH_2CH_3$ and $CH_3OCH_2CH_2CH_3$ are

   (a) Functional isomers
   (b) Metamers
   (c) Chain isomers
   (d) Keto-enol isomers

10. Which of the statements are incorrect about tautomers

    (a) Tautomers are structural isomers

    (b) They exist in equilibrium mixtures

    (c) It is possible in both acidic and basic medium

    (d) Tautomers have independent existence.

Answers for MCQs

1. (a)   2. (a)   3. (b)   4. (a)   5. (c)

6. (a)   7. (b)   8. (a)   9. (b)   10. (a)

Short Answer Questions

1. Draw the structure corresponding to the IUPAC name of 2,4,6-trinitrophenol, 1,3,5-trifluorobenzene, 3-amino-4-methylphenol, 3-chloro-2-phenyl-3-heptene.

2. Draw the structure corresponding to the IUPAC name of 3-chloro-2-phenyl-3-heptene.

2. Write down the IUPAC name of $CH_3COCH_2CH_2CH_2COOH$.

3. Write down the IUPAC name of $CH_3CH(CH_3)COCONHBr$.

4. Write IUPAC names of following organic compounds.

a) [structure: CH_3-CH=CH-$CH(NH_2)$-$COOH$]

b) [structure: ketone and ester with OCH_3]

c) [structure: alkene]

d) [structure: pentane chain]

e) NCCH$_2$CHCN
       |
      CHO

f) [structure: branched alkane]

g) CH$_3$CH$_2$CCH$_2$CH$_3$
         ‖
         CH$_2$

h) CHO
   |
   COOH

Long Answer Questions

1. In the structures given below identify the following:

   I. CH_3—CH_2—CH_2—CH_2—OH

   II. CH_3—CH_2—CH—CH_3
                      |
                     OH

   III.
   $$CH_3-\underset{\underset{OH}{|}}{\overset{\overset{CH_3}{|}}{C}}-CH_3$$

   IV. CH_3—CH—CH_2—OH
                |
               CH_3

   V. CH_3—CH_2—O—CH_2—CH_3

   VI. CH_3—O—CH_2—CH_2—CH_3

   VII. CH_3—O—CH—CH_3
                    |
                   CH_3

1. Which of the above compounds form pairs of metamers?

2. Identify the pairs of compounds which are functional group isomers.

3. Identify the pairs of compounds that represents position isomerism.

4. Identify the pairs of compounds that represents chain isomerism.

5. What do you mean by structural isomers? Discuss the various type of structural isomers with its examples.

Alkanes, Alkanes and Conjugated Dienes

Alkanes are aliphatic hydrocarbons having formula written in generalized form i.e. C_nH_{2n+2} where the number of carbon atoms is denoted by n. In alkanes, carbon atom contains only single covalent bonds (between carbon and hydrogen). The alicyclic saturated hydrocarbons are called paraffins which is derived from Latin word, parum affins which means little affinity) because they have a low reactivity to most reagents, including acids, alkalis, oxidizing and reducing agents. However, alkanes exhibit a few reactions under extreme circumstances, such as free radical chain halogenation, nitration, sulphonation, and pyrolysis, when exposed to high temperatures and pressure.

Carbon chain	IUPAC name	General Formula
1	Methane	CH_4
2	Ethane-	C_2H_6
3	Propane	C_3H_8
4	Butane	C_4H_{10}
5	Pentane	C_5H_{12}
6	Hexane	C_6H_{14}
10	Decane	$C_{10}H_{22}$
20	Eicosane	$C_{20}H_{22}$
30	Triacontane	$C_{30}H_{62}$

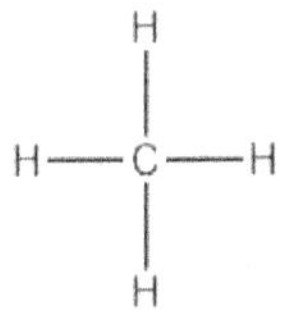

or

CH_4

Methane

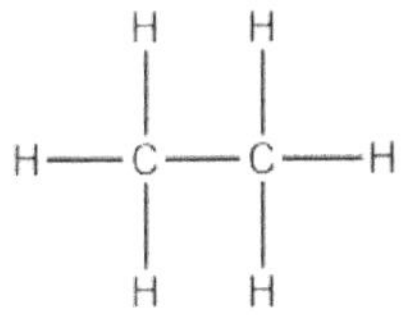

or

C_2H_6

Ethane

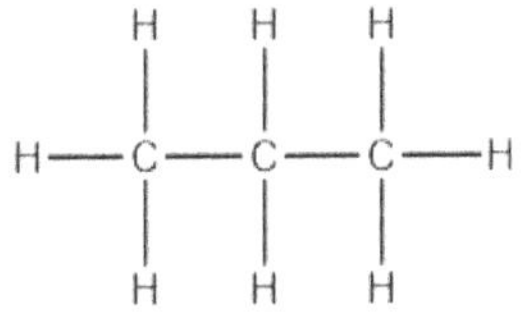

or

C_3H_8

Propane

Structure of Alkanes

The structure of alkanes can be explained by Electronic Theory of valency and the concept of hybridization of carbon, the structure of methane and ethane are explained as follows:

Carbon contains four unpaired valence electrons as illustrated below:

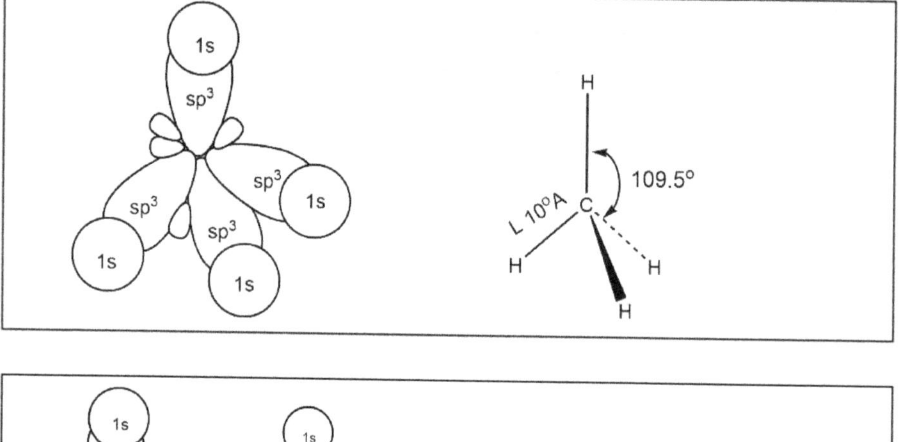

Ground state   Excited state   Equal energy states after sp^3
electronic configuration of C   electronic configuration of C   hybridisation

It may be noted that each carbon in alkanes is sp^{3}hybridised. These sp^3 hybridised carbon use their four half-filled sp^3-hybridised orbitals pointing towards the corners of a tetrahedron to form sigma bonds. Each carbon atom of alkanes contains four bonding orbitals which is used to make covalent bond with similar orbitals of other carbon atoms or 1s orbitals of hydrogen atoms resulting in bond angle of 109°28'between any two adjacent bonds.

In case of methane, four sigma covalent bonds are formed by overlapping of 1s orbitals of four hydrogens with four sp^3 orbitals of carbon.

In the same way, in case of ethane and higher members of alkanes, the relative arrangement of bonds is always tetrahedral. Alkanes have just single covalent carbon-carbon and carbon-hydrogen bonds with bond lengths of 154pm and 112pm, respectively.

Different carbon atoms in alkanes:

Four types of carbon atoms are present in alkanes which are as follows:

(i) Primary carbon atom (1°): Primary carbon atoms are carbon atoms that are directly bound to one or more carbon atoms.

(ii) Secondary carbon atom (2°): A secondary carbon atom is a carbon atom that is directly connected to two other carbon atoms.

(iii) Tertiary carbon atoms (3°): A tertiary carbon atom is one that is directly connected to three other carbon atoms.

(iv) Quaternary carbon atoms (4°): Quaternary carbon atoms are carbon atoms that are directly linked to four other carbon atoms.

Consider an example:

$$
\begin{array}{ccccc}
 & & & \overset{\displaystyle 1^{\cdot}}{CH_3} & \\
 \overset{\displaystyle 1^{\cdot}}{CH_3} & - & \underset{H_2}{\overset{\displaystyle 2^{\cdot}}{C}} & - & \underset{4^{\cdot}}{C} & - & \overset{\displaystyle 1^{\cdot}}{CH_3} \\
 & & & \underset{\displaystyle 1^{\cdot}}{CH_3} &
\end{array}
$$

Four primary carbons (connected to only one carbon atom), one secondary carbon (connected to two carbon atoms), and one quaternary carbon atom make up the above molecule (attached to four carbon atoms).

Physical Properties of Alkanes

Because alkanes have covalent C-C and C-H bonds and very low electronegativity between carbon and hydrogen atoms, their physical characteristics are determined by intermolecular forces of attraction, also known as van der Waals forces. The region of contact between neighbouring molecules determines the amount of van der Waals forces. The following are some of the physical characteristics of alkanes:

Boiling Points: The straight chain alkanes' first four members (C1-C4) are gases, the following thirteen are liquids (C5-C17), and the upper members (C18 onwards) are colourless waxy solids. As the number of carbon atoms rises, the boiling temperatures of n-alkanes climb inexorably. The boiling point rises by 20-30K when a carbon atom or a CH_2 group is added.

The constant increase in the boiling temperatures of straight chain alkanes with increasing carbon content can be explained by intermolecular forces of attraction. These forces act on the surface of molecules, and their magnitude grows as the size of the molecules grows. As a result, the magnitude of van der Waal's forces of attraction becomes stronger, raising the boiling point.

The boiling point of the branched chain isomer of isomeric alkanes is lower than that of the corresponding n-alkanes. As branching increases, the surface area of the branched isomer diminishes. Because the surface area of these molecules is smaller, the van der Waals forces of attraction that work between them are weaker, needing less energy to overcome. As a result, the boiling temperatures of branched chain isomers are lower than those of comparable n-alkanes.

The boiling temperatures of n-pentane, iso-pentane, and neo-pentane, for example, are 309, 301, and 282.5 degrees Celsius, respectively.

1. Melting points—Alkanes' melting points, like their boiling temperatures, rise as the carbon number rises, but the increase is not uniform.

   When traveling from an alkane with an odd number of carbon atoms to a higher alkane, the rise in melting point is substantially more than when traveling from an alkane with an even number of carbon atoms to a higher alkane. Alkanes produce zig-zag chains rather than straight chains, which explains this. In alkanes with an even number of carbon atoms, the terminal methyl groups are on opposing ends of the zig-zag chain. The terminal methyl groups of n-alkanes with an odd number of carbon atoms are placed on the same side of the chains as shown below:

   n-Hexane
   (even number of carbon atoms)

   n-Heptane
   (odd number of carbon atoms)

   Alkanes with an even number of carbon atoms are found to fit tightly together in the crystal structure, but alkanes with an odd number of carbon atoms do not. As a result, the energy needed to break the crystal structure and melt alkanes with an even number of carbon atoms is higher than the energy needed to shatter the crystal structure with an odd number of carbon atoms.

Hydrocarbon (Straight chain isomers)	C_3H_8	C_4H_{10}	C_5H_{12}	C_6H_{14}	C_7H_{16}	C_8H_{18}
Melting points(K)	85.9	138	143.3	179	182.5	216.2

2. Specific gravity—Alkane specific gravities grow with increasing molecular weights, but stabilize at 0.8. As a result, alkanes all have a lower density than water.

3. Solubility- When it comes to solubility, the basic rule is that "like dissolves like." Alkanes are non-polar in nature because the electronegativities of carbon and hydrogen are virtually similar. Alkanes are soluble in non-polar solvents such as ether, benzene, and so on, but insoluble in polar solvents such as water, alcohol, and so on, due to their non-polar character.

Natural sources of Alkanes:

Alkanes can be found in nature in the following places:

The two primary commercial sources of alkanes are petroleum (crude oil) and natural gas. Plants and creatures that have been buried for a long time are created by high temperature and pressure, as well as anaerobic conditions. Petroleum, which is found naturally underneath the earth's surface, is used to create a mixture of alkanes. Furthermore, natural gas emitted from petroleum fields and fuel gases have lower alkane levels. Because alkanes are saturated hydrocarbons with single bonds, they do not readily react. Alkanes will react with oxygen if given enough Activation Energy. Alkanes create carbon dioxide and water as a result of this highly exothermic process, making them suitable as fuels.

Methods of Preparation of Alkanes

Alkanes are abundantly found in petroleum, hence synthesis of alkanes is rarely carried out in reality. Many alkanes, however, are not found in petroleum, and we must create them in a laboratory. The following are some of the most common ways for preparing alkanes:

1. **From unsaturated hydrocarbons (Sabatier and Senderen's Reactions)-** Alkenes and alkynes are added to hydrogen in the presence of a catalyst such as Raney nickel, platinum, or palladium to create alkanes.

$$C_nH_{2n} + H_2 \xrightarrow[525\text{-}575K]{Ni} C_nH_{2n-2}$$

Alkene

$$CH_2 = CH_2 + H_2 \xrightarrow[525\text{-}575K]{Ni} CH_3 - CH_3$$

Ethylene · · · Ethane

$$C_nH_{2n-2} + 2H_2 \xrightarrow[525\text{-}575K]{Ni} C_nH_{2n-2}$$

Alkyne

$$CH \equiv CH + 2H_2 \xrightarrow[525\text{-}575K]{Ni} CH_3 - CH_3$$

Acetylene · · · Ethane

The use of nickel as a hydrogenation catalyst necessitates a temperature of around 525-575K. When platinum or palladium is utilized as a catalyst, however, the reaction occurs at room temperature.

The disadvantage of this reaction is that it cannot produce methane since the starting alkene or alkyne must have at least two carbon atoms.

2. **From alkyl halides-** The following procedures can be used to convert alkyl halides to alkanes:

I Using the Grignard reagent- Alkyl halides react with magnesium metal in the presence of dry ether to produce alkyl magnesium halide, also known as the Grignard reagent. Alkanes are formed when Grignard reagent reacts with substances containing active hydrogens.

$$CH_3CH_2 - Br + Mg \xrightarrow{dry\ ether} CH_3CH_2 - MgBr$$

Bromoethane · · · Ethylmagnesium bromide

$$CH_3CH_2 - MgBr + H_2O \longrightarrow CH_3CH_3 + Mg(OH)Br$$

Ethylmagnesium bromide · · · Ethane

$$CH_3\!-\!MgI \quad + \quad CH_3OH \quad \longrightarrow \quad CH_4 \; + \; Mg(OCH_3)I$$

Methylmagnesium   methanol   methane
iodide

(i)   **Wurtz reaction-** Alkyl halides on treatment with metallic sodium in the presence of dry diethyl ether, results in the formation of alkane obtained by fusion of two alkyl groups.

$$R\text{-}X \; +2Na \; + X\text{-}R \xrightarrow{\text{dry ether}} R\text{-}R + \; 2NaI$$

Alkyl halide   Alkane

$$CH_3I \; + \; 2Na \; + \; ICH_3 \xrightarrow{\text{dry ether}} CH_3\text{-}CH_3 \; +2NaI$$

Methyl iodide   Ethane

When the reaction takes place between same alkyl halide, a symmetrical alkane with even number of carbon atoms is obtained.

However, during synthesis of unsymmetrical alkane containing three or more carbon atoms, a mixture of mixture of alkyl halides are used. The final product contains a mixture of alkanes.

For example, consider synthesis of propane,

$$CH_3Br \; +2Na \; + \; BrCH_2CH_3 \xrightarrow{\text{dry ether}} CH_3CH_2CH_3 \; +2NaBr$$

Methyl bromide   Ethyl bromide   Propane

In the above reaction propane along with n-butane and ethane are obtained which are difficult to separate out.

The order of reactivity of different alkyl halides in this reaction follows the trend:

Iodides > Bromides > Chlorides

However due to mixture of alkanes obtained when different alkyl halides are used makes this reaction less important because the alkanes belonging to same family have identical physical properties making them quite difficult to separate. This is because the two alkyl halides in react with each other resulting into a mixture of alkanes as illustrated below:

$$CH_3\text{---}I \;+\; 2Na \;+\; I\text{---}CH_2CH_3 \xrightarrow{\text{dry ether}} CH_3\text{---}CH_2CH_3 \;+2NaI$$

Methyliodide   Ethyliodide   Propane

$$CH_3\text{---}I \;+\; 2Na \;+\; I\text{---}CH_3 \xrightarrow{\text{dry ether}} CH_3CH_3 \;+\; 2NaI$$

Ethane

$$CH_3CH_2\text{---}I \;+\; 2Na \;+\; I\text{---}CH_2CH_3 \xrightarrow{\text{dry ether}} CH_3CH_2\text{---}CH_2CH_3 \;+2NaI$$

Butane

Limitations:

(a) One serious drawback of Wurtz reaction is it can be used for the synthesis of only alkanes containing even number of carbon atoms and not for the preparation of unsymmetrical alkanes with odd number of carbon atoms.

(b) It cannot be used for the preparation of methane.

(c) Tert. Butyl halides cannot be used in this reaction.

(ii) Corey- House reaction- In Corey-House reaction alkyl halides react with lithium dialkyl copper to produce alkanes. This method is considered better than Wurtz reaction since both symmetrical and unsymmetrical alkanes can be synthesized by this method.

$$R'\text{-}X \;+\; R_2CuLi \longrightarrow R\text{-}R' \;+\; RCu \;+\; LiX$$

Alkyl halide   lithium   alkane
                 dialkyl copper

For example,

$$CH_3CH_2CH_2Br \;+\; (CH_3)_2CuLi \longrightarrow CH_3CH_2CH_3 \;+\; CH_3Cu \;+\; LiBr$$

n-Butyl bromide   lithium dimethyl copper   n-propane   Methyl copper

(iii) Reduction of Alkyl halides- Alkyl halides are converted to alkanes by direct reduction with chemical reducing agents such as zinc and hydrochloric or with hydrogen in the presence of palladium catalyst or by heating alkyl iodides with hydrogen iodide in the presence of red-hot sealed tube.

$$RX \xrightarrow{\text{Zn/H}^+} RH \;+\; HX$$

Alkyl halide   Alkane

$$CH_3CH_2CH_2CH_2Br \xrightarrow{\text{Zn/H}^-} CH_3CH_2CH_2CH_3 \;+HBr$$

n-Butyl bromide   n-butane

$$C_2H_5I \ + HI \xrightarrow{\text{Red P}} C_2H_6 \ + I_2$$

Ethyl iodide   Ethane

3. From carboxylic acid

(i) Kolbe's electrolytic reaction- In this reaction, concentrated aqueous solution of sodium or potassium salts of monocarboxylic acids is subjected to electrolysis to get alkanes.

$$2RCOONa + 2H_2O \xrightarrow{\text{Electrolysis}} R\!-\!\!-\!R \ + 2NaOH \ + H_2$$

Alkane

The reaction takes place as follows:

$$2RCOONa \rightleftharpoons 2RCOO^- \ + \ 2Na^+$$

Sodium salt of acid

$$2H_2O \rightleftharpoons 2H^+ \ + \ 2OH^-$$

At the anode

$$2RCOO^- \longrightarrow 2RCOO+2e^- \longrightarrow R\text{-}R \ + \ 2CO_2$$

Alkane

At the cathode

$$2H+ 2e\text{-} \longrightarrow H_2$$

When compared to Na^+ ions, H^+ ions have a lower discharge potential. As a result, H^+ ions are released at the cathode, releasing H_2, while Na^+ ions stay in solution.

This is an excellent way to make ethane and other higher alkanes with an even number of carbon atoms.

This approach will not produce methane.

(ii) Monocarboxylic acid decarboxylation- When sodium salts of monocarboxylic acids are heated with soda lime (NaOH+ CaO), carbon dioxide is liberated from the carboxylic group.

$$RCOONa + NaOH \xrightarrow{\text{CaO}} RH \ + \ Na_2CO_3$$

Sodium salt of acid   Alkane

$$CH_3COONa + NaOH \longrightarrow CH_4 + Na_2CO_3$$

Sodium acetate   Methane

Chemical Reactions of Alkanes

Alkanes are saturated hydrocarbons with only strong C-H and C-C sigma bonds, making them very reactive. Because alkanes are non-reactive, they do not react with acids, alkalis, or oxidizing or reducing agents in normal circumstances. However, alkanes do conduct a few reactions at extreme circumstances, the majority of which involve replacements via the free radical chain mechanism.

The following are some of the most important alkane chemical reactions:

1. **Halogenation-** One or more hydrogen atoms in an alkane are replaced by halogen atoms in this process.

   $F_2 > Cl_2 > Br_2 > I_2$ is the order of halogen reactivity.

   - Alkanes react aggressively with the fluorine radical, which is the most reactive of the halogen free radicals. The iodine radical, on the other hand, is the least reactive of the halogen radicals and has no interaction with alkane.

   - When compared to chlorination, bromination occurs at a significantly slower rate. Furthermore, the activation energy required to abstract a hydrogen atom by a bromine radical is about 4.5 times that required to abstract a hydrogen atom by a chlorine radical.

   - Experiments on chlorination and bromination include reacting an alkane with chlorine or bromine in the presence of light or at high temperatures (525-673K). When methane gets chlorinated in the presence of UV radiation, for example, the hydrogens in the methane are replaced by chlorine atoms, as seen below:

$$CH_4 + Cl_2 \longrightarrow CH_3Cl + HCl$$

Methane   Chloromethane

$$CH_3Cl + Cl_2 \longrightarrow CH_2Cl_2 + HCl$$

Dichloromethane

$$CH_2Cl_2 + Cl_2 \longrightarrow CHCl_3 + HCl$$

Trichloromethane

$$CHCl_3 + Cl_2 \longrightarrow CCl_4 + HCl$$

Tetrachloromethane

Mechanism

A. Chlorination and Bromination-Halogenation of alkanes occurs through free radicals involving chain reaction mechanism. The reaction takes place in the following steps:

(i) X—X $\longrightarrow$ $\dot{X} + \dot{X}$ (Chain inititating step)

(ii) R—$H + \dot{X}$ $\longrightarrow$ $\cdot R + H$—X

  alkane   (Chain propogarting step)

  $\dot{R} + X$—X $\longrightarrow$ R—$X + \dot{X}$

(iii) $\dot{X} + \dot{X}$ $\longrightarrow$ X_2 (Chain terminating step)

(i) **Chain Initiating Step:** The halogen molecule takes up energy either from ultra-violet light or from heat to form halogen atoms or free radicals by homolysis.

(ii) **Chain propagating step**: The free radical X· collides with an alkane molecule to form alkyl free radical. The reaction is exothermic. The alkyl free radical then attacks with halogen molecule to form alkyl halide and X· free radical.

The two steps involved in the chain propagating steps are repeated again and again forming more and more alkyl halide molecules. Consider reaction of methyl halide with halogen free radical, it is observed that di, tri and tetra substituted products are also obtained as follows:

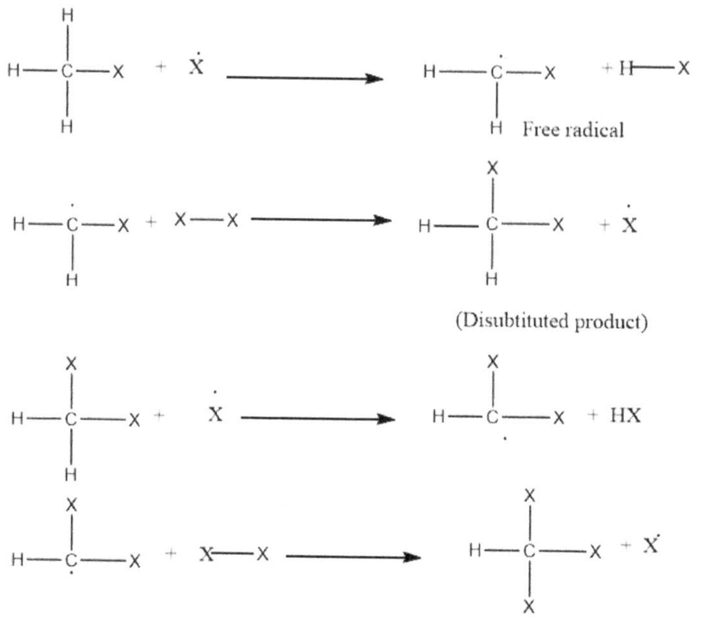

(Disubtituted product)

(Trisubstituted product)

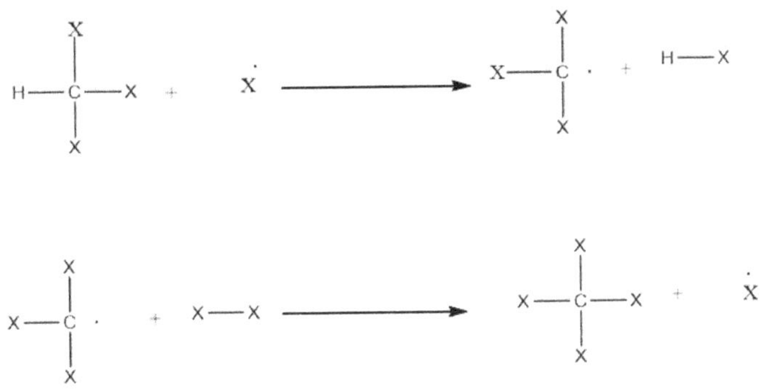

(tetrasubstituted product)

(iii) Chain terminating step- At the end, the reaction stops by mutually combining the free radicals.

$$\dot{X} \ + \ \dot{X} \longrightarrow X_2$$

Halogen molecule

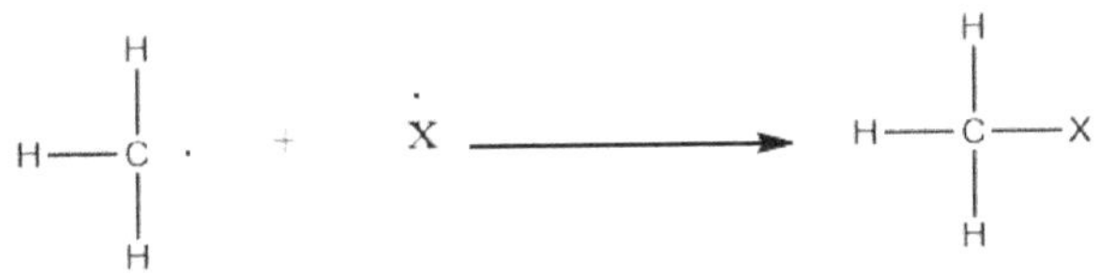

Methyl halide

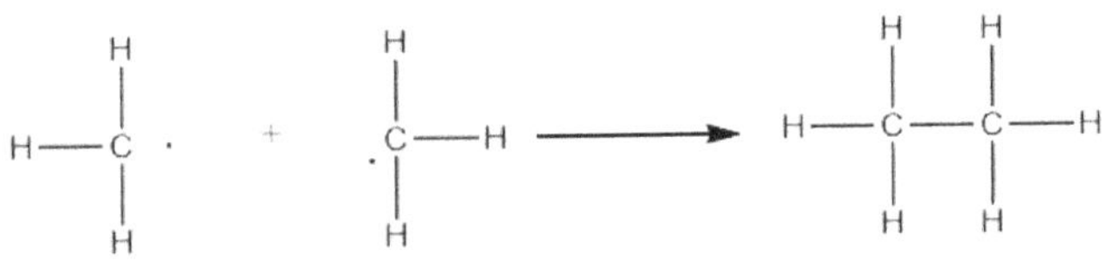

Ethane

Selectivity of Bromination- Bromination of methane is slower than chlorination although bromine atoms dissociate into atoms more rapidly than dissociation of chlorine molecules because the following steps involving the dissociation of molecules(X_2) into atoms ($2X\cdot$), therefore, ΔH is equal to $E_{act.}$

$$Cl-Cl \longrightarrow 2\dot{C}l \qquad \Delta H = +242.5 \text{ kJ mol}^{-1}$$

$$Br-Br \longrightarrow 2\dot{B}r \qquad \Delta H = +192.5 \text{ kJ mol}^{-1}$$

Chlorine with largest E_{act} (242.5KJ mol^{-1}) should dissociate more slowly whereas bromine with smallest E_{act} (192.5KJ mol^{-1}) should dissociate rapidly. Overall bromination is slower than chlorination because the second step which involves the abstraction of hydrogen atom and formation of alkyl free radical has value of E_{act} to be 17kJ and 75kJ respectively for reactions involving chlorine and bromine atoms and hence the overall rate of reaction becomes slower for bromination as compared to chlorination.

Bromine is less reactive but more selective as compared to chlorine. The chlorination of n-butane gives 28% 1-chlorobutane and 72% of 2-chlorobutane. However, the percentage of the two isomers in the bromination are 2% and 98% respectively. Thus, the product of bromination is almost 2-bromobutane with a negligible amount of 1-bromobutane. Clearly bromination is preferred to chlorination in the preparation of alkyl halide.

It can be understood by considering the relative rate of abstraction of the different hydrogen atoms in the chlorination and bromination of alkanes. In the chlorination, the relative rate of abstraction of hydrogen atoms by chlorine atoms is 1:3.8. Thus, the percentages of 1-chlorobutane and 2-chlorobutane.

$$\frac{1-\text{chlorobutane}}{2-\text{chlorobutane}} = \frac{\text{No. of } 1°-H}{\text{No. of } 2°-H} \times \frac{\text{Reactivity of } 1°-H}{\text{Reactivity of } 2°-H}$$

$$= \frac{6}{4} \times \frac{1}{3.8} = \frac{6}{15.2} = \frac{28\%}{72\%}$$

In the bromination, the relative rates of abstraction of the primary and secondary hydrogen atoms are in the ratio of 1:82. Thus, the relative percentages of bromobutanes are:

$$\frac{1-\text{Bromobutane}}{2-\text{Bromobutane}} = \frac{\text{No. of } 1°-H}{\text{No. of } 2°-H} \times \frac{\text{Reactivity of } 1°-H}{\text{Reactivity of } 2°-H}$$

$$= \frac{6}{4} \times \frac{1}{82} = \frac{6}{164} = \frac{2\%}{98\%}$$

B. Fluorination of alkanes- Fluorine radical reacts very violently with alkanes resulting in the cleavage of C-C and C-H bonds. This can be explained by considering the bond dissociation energies of various species involved in the chain initiation and propagation.

$$F\text{-}F \longrightarrow 2\,F \qquad \Delta H = +159kJ$$

$$F + H\text{-}CH_3 \longrightarrow CH_3 + H\text{-}F \qquad \Delta H = -133kJ$$

$$CH_3 + F\text{-}F \longrightarrow CH_3\text{-}F + F \qquad \Delta H = -292kJ$$

From the above equations, it is clear that overall fluorination reaction is highly exothermic and the release of such a huge amount of energy explains why fragmentation of alkanes takes place.

C. Iodination of alkanes- The I-I bond among the halogens is the weakest due to the least value of bond dissociation energy (151.0kJ mol^{-1}). But still the iodination is very less common as compared to chlorination or bromination. This is due to the fact that iodine free radical formed is to attack alkane molecule in the chain propagating step. This requires a very high activation energy. Consequently, iodination is least common in the halogenation of alkanes. Hence, the direct iodination of alkane fails to product an alkyl iodide. This is because the by-product HI reduces iodoalkane back to alkane.

Hence, strong oxidizing agents like iodic acid, nitric acid or HgO are used which destroys the HI and prevent the reversibility of the reaction.

$$CH_3\text{-}H + I \longrightarrow CH_3 + H\text{-}I \qquad \Delta H = +138kJ\ mol^{-1}$$

Nitric acid used in the reaction reacts with HI produced and hence help in moving the reaction in forward direction.

$$5HI + HIO_3 \longrightarrow 3H_2O + 3I_2$$

2. **Nitration of alkane-** Replacement of hydrogen atom of alkane with nitro group (-NO$_2$) is called nitration of alkane. The reaction takes place by two methods:

   (i) **Liquid phase nitration-** Higher alkane when heated with fuming nitric acid at 413K under pressure results in replacement of one hydrogen atom with nitro group.

$$C_6H_{13}H + HONO_2 \longrightarrow C_6H_{13}NO_2 + H_2O$$
$$\text{Hexane} \qquad\qquad \text{Nitric acid} \qquad\qquad \text{Nitrohexane}$$

   (ii) **Vapour phase nitration-** Nitration of lower members of alkanes is carried out in vapour phase by heating a gaseous mixture of hydrocarbon with nitric acid at 673-773K.

$$CH_3\text{-}H + HO\text{-}NO_2 \longrightarrow CH_3NO_2 + H_2O$$
$$\text{Nitromethane}$$
$$C_2H_5\text{-}H + HO\text{-}NO_2 \longrightarrow C_2H_5\text{-}NO_2 + H_2O$$
$$\text{Nitroethane}$$

3. **Sulphonation of alkane-** This process involves the replacement of hydrogen atom of alkanes with sulphonic acid group(-SO$_3$H) by heating higher alkanes with fuming sulphuric acid.

$$C_6H_{13}H + HOSO_3H \xrightarrow{\text{Heat}} C_6H_{13}SO_3H + H_2O$$

   (i) **Complete combustion or complete oxidation:** Alkanes burn in excess of air or oxygen to produce carbon dioxide and water.

$$CH_4 + 2O_2 \longrightarrow CO_2(g) + 2H_2O(g)$$
$$\text{Methane}$$

$$C_2H_6(g) + 7/2\ O_2(g) \longrightarrow 2CO_2 + 3H_2O$$
$$\text{Ethane}$$

Alkanes are useful fuels because of the huge amounts of heat released during burning.

(ii) Incomplete combustion- When combustion occurs in unsufficient air or oxygen, soot or carbon black is obtained, that is used to make inks and polishes.

(iii) Regulated combustion - When heated in a controlled supply of air or oxygen at high temperatures under high pressure in the presence of a catalyst such as copper or molybdenum oxide, alkanes are oxidized to alcohols and aldehydes

$$2CH_4 + O_2 \xrightarrow[120 \text{ atom. } 475K]{\text{Cu tube}} 2CH_3OH$$

Methane   Methyl alcohol

$$CH_4 + O_2 \xrightarrow{\text{Molybdenum oxide}} HCHO + H_2O$$

Methane   Formaldehyde

4. Isomerization of alkanes- Straight chain alkanes are converted into isomeric branched chain alkanes during alkane isomerization.

Example: On treating butane with aluminium chloride in the presence of dry HCl gas at 573K under about 35 atmospheric pressure, 2-methyl propane is produced.

$$CH_3-CH_2-CH_2-CH_3 \xrightarrow[\text{HCl gas}]{AlCl_3} CH_3-\underset{\underset{CH_3}{|}}{CH}-CH_3$$

n-butane   2-methylpropane
                                                     (isobutane)

Uses of Paraffins

➤ Paraffin wax is used as a component in lotions, pastes, creams, lipsticks, and as a tablet coating to preserve the surface of tablets, postpone the release of their contents, and boost their shine. To facilitate handling, transport, and dispensing of fertiliser, the fertiliser industry employs paraffins and special mixtures as anti-caking agents.

➤ In medicine, liquid paraffin is most commonly used as a paediatric laxative and is a popular treatment for constipation and encopresis.

➤ It can be used on capsules and tablets as a release agent, binder, or lubricant.

➤ Paraffin is used as a moisture repellent and to ensure the rigidity and impermeability of the cupboards.

➤ Paraffin acts as a barrier against moisture, microorganisms, and odours, as well as preserving the aroma and flavour of the wrapped product.

➢ It can also be found in matches, the textile industry, explosives, rubbers, grafts, corks, skiing and surfing equipment, and electrical and electronic applications, to name a few.

➢ People suffering from the following conditions may benefit from the use of paraffin wax to help relieve pain in their hands:

➢ Paraffin is water resistant by nature. Waterproofing may be done with paraffin wax coatings on a range of goods, including matches, wood, and bottles.

➢ Because paraffin wax candles burn cleaner and more consistently than tallow candles, they were first used to replace them. Because it is colourless and odourless, paraffin wax is ideal for making custom scented candles. Paraffin candles can also be used.

Alkenes Introduction

Alkenes are unsaturated acyclic hydrocarbons containing a double bond between carbon and carbon. The typical chemical formula for alkenes is $CnHn$, where n is the number of carbon atoms. Lower alkenes like ethene, propene, and others make oily compounds when exposed to halogens like chlorine and bromine, therefore they're called olefins (Greek: olefiant = oil creating). A carbon-carbon double bond exists in alkene molecules. The C=C bond is made up of one strong sigma bond and one weak pi bond. The electrons in the pi bond are more exposed, which increases reactivity. In other words, alkenes are more chemically reactive than alkanes due to the presence of the pi bond, which is formed by the sideways overlapping of atomic orbitals.

Number of carbon atoms	Structure	IUPAC name
2	$CH_2=CH_2$	Ethene
3	$CH_3CH=CH_2$	Propene
4	$CH_3CH_2=CHCH_3$	But-1-ene
4	$CH_3CH=CHCH_3$	But-2-ene
5	$CH_3CH_2CH_2CH=CH_2$	Pent-1-ene
5	$CH_3CH_2CH=CHCH_3$	Pent-2-ene
6	$CH_3CH_2CH_2CH_2CH=CH_2$	Hex-1-ene
6	$CH_3CH_2CH_2CH=CHCH_3$	Hex-2-ene

Structure of Alkenes

Alkene molecules are distinguished by the presence of a carbon-carbon double bond in their molecules. The doubly bound carbon is undergoing sp^2 hybridisation, as demonstrated here: The two carbon atoms of ethene that are connected by a double bond employ three equivalent sp^2 hybridized orbitals and an unhybridized p-orbital of both carbon atoms to create this molecule. The overlap of a sp^2 orbital of one carbon with a sp^2 orbital of the second carbon produces one of ethylene's carbon-carbon bonds. The overlap of one of each carbon's remaining hybridised orbitals with the 1s orbital of a hydrogen forms each of the four carbon hydrogen bonds. The connections formed by orbitals overlapping along their axes are known as sigma bonds. In addition, each carbon atom's three sp^2 orbitals are in the same plane, and all carbon and hydrogen atoms in ethene are co-planar. As a result, ethene is a flat molecule with each carbon atom at the center of a triangle and two hydrogen atoms and the other carbon atom at the corners, as seen below:

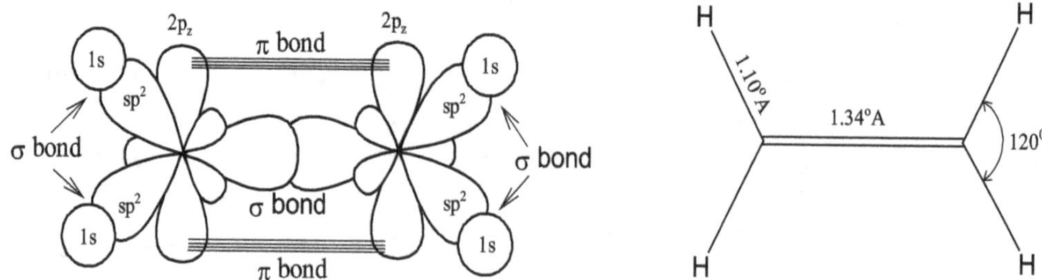

An unhybridized half-filled p-orbital at right angles to the plane containing the carbon and hydrogen sigma electron framework generates the remaining pi bond. The unhybridized p-orbitals of the two carbons overlap sideways to create a carbon-carbon double bond. The weak pi is made up of two electron clouds, one above the other (due to the fact that overlapping happens only to a minor level in its formation). The sigma bond between carbon atoms has a strength of 398kJ mol^{-1}, while the pi bond has a strength of 284kJ mol^{-1}. The carbon-carbon double bond in ethene is indisputably stronger than the carbon-carbon single bond in ethane (368kJ mol^{-1}).

The carbon-carbon double bond distance in ethene is 134pm, which is less than the single bond distance. Because a double bond is made up of an additional pi bond generated by the sideways overlapping of carbon atom p-orbitals, the carbon atoms are brought closer together.

Furthermore, the sp^2 orbital of carbon used to make a carbon-carbon double bond is smaller than the sp^3 orbital used to make a carbon-carbon single bond.

Rotation around the C=C bond is hampered.

Isomerism Exhibited by Alkenes

A single bond and a pi bond make up the carbon-carbon double bond in ethene. Unhybridized p-orbitals of carbon atoms overlap above and below the plane of the atoms to form the pi bond. The additional pi link makes rotation around the carbon-carbon double bond difficult, and it can only happen if the pi bond breaks down, which needs roughly 284kJmol-1, which isn't accessible at normal temperature.

Because of the hindered rotation around the carbon-carbon double bond, the relative positions of groups attached to doubly bonded carbon atoms are fixed. As a result, alkenes exhibit geometrical isomerism, which implies they can exist in two different isomeric forms with different relative distributions of groups in space around the double bond.

The prefixes "cis" and "trans" come from Latin, respectively, and indicate "this side of" and "the other side of." In chemistry, cis refers to functional groups on the same side of the carbon chain, whereas trans refers to functional groups on the other side.

2-Butene, for example, can have the following two forms: (cis and trans).

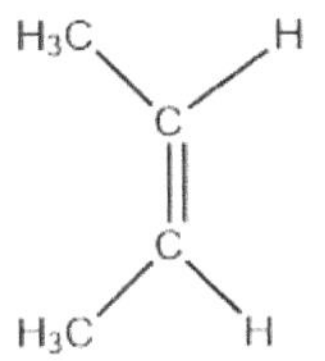

Cis-2-butene

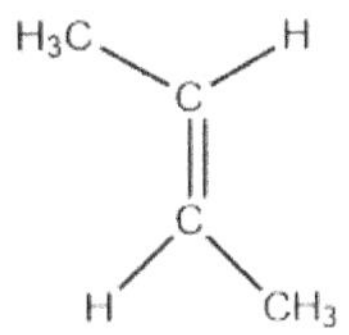

trans-2-butene

Relative Stabilities of Alkenes

The heat of hydrogenation is used to determine alkene relative stabilities. The heat of hydrogenation is the amount of heat emitted when one mole of an unsaturated molecule is entirely hydrogenated. The isomer of an alkene with more heat of hydrogenation than the other isomer is less stable than the other isomer because the higher the heat of hydrogenation of an alkene, the higher the energy content and hence the less stable it is. As a result of the heat of hydrogenation of various alkenes, the following conclusions may be drawn:

(i)   Because the two larger substituent groups are widely apart in the trans isomer relative to the cis isomer, a cis alkene is somewhat less stable than the trans isomer in the case of dialkyl derivatives of ethene that exist as geometrical isomers. As a result, the trans-isomer has less crowding and van der Waals strain than the cis isomer, and hence is more stable. As an example,

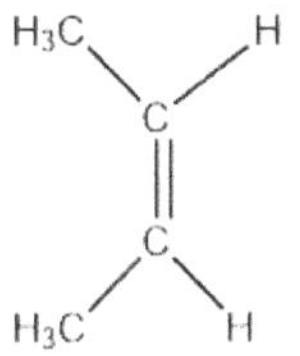

Cis-2-butene

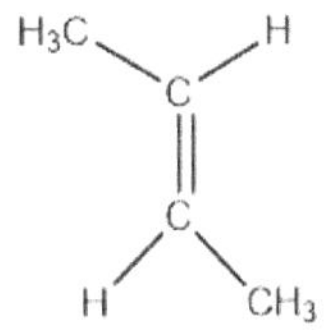

trans-2-butene

As the van der Waals strain increases, the stability decreases. Because there is less van der Waals strain, the system is more stable.

(ii)   The alkene becomes more stable as the number of alkyl groups attached to the doubly linked carbon atoms increases.

As a result, relative stabilities are in the following order: $R_2C{=}CR_2 > R_2C{=}CRH > R_2{=}CH_2 > RCH{=}CHR > RCH{=}CH_2 > CH_2{=}CH_2$.

Hyperconjugation can be used to describe the preceding arrangement. The more alkyl groups attached to doubly bounded carbon atoms, the more hyperconjugating structures are formed, and hence the alkene's stability increases.

Physical Properties of Alkenes

Alkenes have the following physical properties:

1. **Physical state:** The first three alkenes are gases, followed by fourteen liquids, and finally solids. This is because the van der Waal forces of attraction between molecules increase as molecular weight increases. The remaining constituents, with the exception of ethene, which has a mild pleasant odor, are colorless and odourless.

2. **Boiling points:** As the number of carbon atoms rises, the boiling points of alkenes rise in a predictable pattern. Because van der Waal's forces are lower for members with reduced surface area, branched chain alkenes have lower boiling temperatures than isomeric alkenes.

3. **Polarity:** Symmetrical alkenes' trans-isomers are non-polar in nature. Unsymmetrical alkenes, on the other hand, and cis-isomers of symmetrical alkenes are polar and have tiny dipole moments.

Non-polar   Slightly polar

Because they are more polar than their trans isomers, cis alkenes have somewhat higher boiling points. However, because cis isomers are unsymmetrical, they are not as tightly packed in the solid state and so have lower melting temperatures than trans isomers.

4. **Solubility:** Alkenes are water insoluble but easily soluble in organic solvents including benzene, ether, and carbon tetrachloride.

5. **Melting points and specific gravities:** Alkenes have a systematic gradient of melting points and specific gravities. However, alkenes have a maximum specific gravity of 0.8, similar to alkanes. As a result, alkenes are all lighter than water.

Preparations of Alkenes

Alkenes are prepared in a variety of ways.

1. Alkenes may be made from alkyl halides by heating them in an alcoholic potassium hydroxide solution. A halogen acid molecule is eliminated from the equation. The dehydrogenation reaction is the name for this process.

$$C_nH_{2n+1}X + KOH \xrightarrow{\text{Alcohol}} C_nH_{2n} + KX + H_2O$$

Alkyl halide   Alkene

Ethyl bromide $+$ KOH (alc.) $\longrightarrow$ $H_2C=CH_2$ + KBr + H_2O (ethene)

n-propyl bromide $+$ KOH (alc.) $\longrightarrow$ $CH_3-CH=CH_2$ + KBr + H_2O (Propylene)

Above reaction called as the elimination reaction because it involves the removal of a halogen atom and a hydrogen atom from a beta-carbon close to one that is losing the halogen.

Mechanism: The mechanism involves a single step bimolecular elimination process. The nucleophilic OH^- removes the proton from β-carbon atom. Simultaneously, the halide ion is lost from the α-carbon leading to the formation of alkene.

$$\text{slow} \quad RHC=CH_2 + H_2O + X^-$$

Alkene

Nucleophile (OH^-)

The cleavage of C-H and C-X bonds requires energy and this comes from:

- The formation of bond between the abstracted proton (H^+) and hydroxide ion (OH^-).
- Formation of π- bond which supplies about $284 kJmol^{-1}$ of energy.
- The energy of solvation of the halide ion.

Orientation/ Regioselectivity:

(i) In some cases, dehydrohalogenation yields single alkene.

$$CH_3CH_2CH_2CH_2Br \xrightarrow{\text{alc. KOH}} CH_3CH_2CH=CH_2 + KBr + H_2O$$

1-bromobutane   But-1-ene

$$CH_3 - CH = CH - CH_3$$

But-2-ene (80%)

$$CH_3CH_2CH-CH_3 \xrightarrow[\text{heat}]{\text{KOH (alc)}}$$

Br

$$CH_3 - CH_2 - CH = CH_2$$

But-1-ene (20%)

2-Bromobutane

The formation of but-2-ene as the primary product follows Saytzeff's rule, which stipulates that the dehydrohalogenation process produces a more strongly substituted alkene with fewer hydrogen atoms on the doubly linked carbon atoms.

Dehydration of alcohols: Alcohols are dehydrated to generate alkenes when heated with sulphuric acid or phosphoric acid, or when their vapours are passed over heated alumina (Lewis acid).

$$CH_3CH_2OH \xrightarrow[\text{443K}]{\text{96\% H}_2\text{SO}_4} CH_2 = CH_2 \quad + \quad H_2O$$

Ethyl alcohol   ethylene

$$HO - \underset{\underset{CH_3}{|}}{\overset{\overset{CH_3}{|}}{C}} - CH_3 \xrightarrow[\text{355K}]{\text{20\% H}_2\text{SO}_4} CH_3 - \underset{\underset{CH_3}{|}}{C} = CH_2 \quad + \quad H_2O$$

tert-butyl alcohol   2-methylpropene

The acidic dehydration of alcohols is a unimolecular elimination reaction (i.e., E1) that is carried out using concentrated sulphuric acid when heated. An alkene is generated as a result of the elimination of a water molecule.

The order of reactivity of alcohols towards dehydration is:

Tertiary > Secondary > Primary

Mechanism: The acidic dehydration of alcohols proceeds in the following steps:

(i) Protonation of alcohol

$$H_2SO_4 \rightleftharpoons H^+ + HSO_4^-$$

$$CH_3CH_2-OH + H^+ \longrightarrow CH_3CH_2-\overset{\oplus}{O}-H$$
$$\underset{H}{|}$$

Protonated ethyl alcohol

(ii) Loss of water molecule

$$CH_3CH_2-\overset{\oplus}{\underset{\underset{H}{|}}{O}}-H \xrightarrow{\text{slow}} CH_3\overset{\oplus}{C}H_2 + H_2O$$

(iii) Alkene formation:
The carbocation formed in step (ii) loses a proton from β–carbon to form alkene.

$$H-\overset{\overset{H}{|}}{\underset{\underset{H}{|}}{C}}-\overset{\overset{\oplus}{}}{\underset{\underset{H}{|}}{C}}-H + HSO_4^- \rightleftharpoons H_2C=CH_2 + H_2SO_4$$

Regioselectivity in alcohol dehydration: When isomeric alkenes are possible during dehydration of alcohols, the more stable i.e., highly substituted alkene is the major product. This is known as Saytzeff's rule.

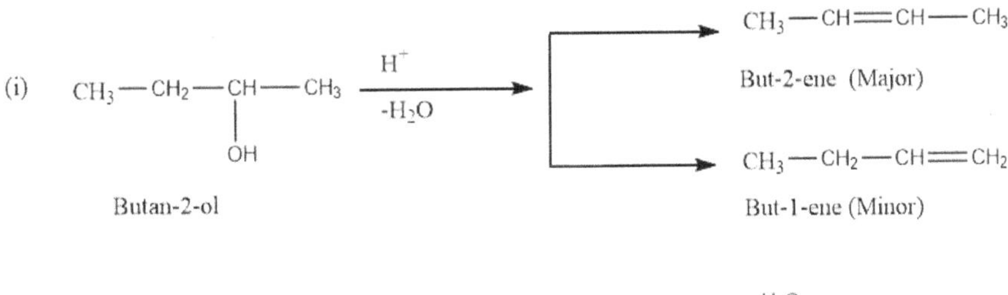

2. **By dehalogenation of vicinal dihalides:** Vicinal halide is a compound having halogens on adjacent carbon atoms. When vic-dihalides are heated with zinc dust in ethyl alcohol, alkenes are obtained.

$$R-CH-CH_2 \ + \ Zn \ \xrightarrow[\text{heat}]{\text{alcohol}} \ R-\underset{H}{C}=CH_2 \ +ZnBr_2$$

Br   Br

vic-dihalide

$$H_3C-CH-CH_2 \ + \ Zn \ \xrightarrow[\text{heat}]{\text{alcohol}} \ CH_3-CH=CH_2 \ + \ ZnBr_2$$

Br   Br

1,2-Dibromopropane   Propene

3. **By partial reduction of alkynes**: Catalytic hydrogenation of alkynes to alkenes is faster than catalytic hydrogenation of alkenes to alkanes. Therefore, by using a specific catalyst, it is possible to stop reduction at the alkene stage. Also, alkenes show geometrical show geometrical isomerism, alkynes can be reduced to give cis- or trans- alkenes depending upon the nature of the catalyst used.

Catalytic reduction of alkynes in the presence of palladium supported over $CaCO_3$ or $BaSO_4$ and palladium supported over $PbCO_3$, S or quinoline (Lindlar's catalyst) predominantly gives cis-alkenes. However, if alkynes are reduced with sodium in liquid ammonia (Birch reduction), trans alkenes are the major products.

Thus,

$$CH_3-C\equiv C-CH_3$$

But-2-yne

H_2——$Pd/CaCO_3$ | $Na/liq.NH_3$

(Lindlar's catalyst) (Birch reduction)

cis-But-2-ene   trans-But-2-ene

4. **Kolbe's electrolytic reaction**: Alkenes are produced by electrolysis of saturated dicarboxylic acid sodium or potassium salts.

For example,

$$CH_2COOK \atop CH_2COOK \quad + \quad 2H_2O \quad \xrightarrow{Electrolysis} \quad {CH_2 \atop \| \atop CH_2} \quad + \quad 2CO_2 \quad + \quad H_2 \quad + \quad 2KOH$$

Pot. succinate   Ethene

$$CH_2COOK \atop CH_2COOK \quad \xrightarrow{Ionisation} \quad {CH_2COO^- \atop CH_2COO^-} \quad + \quad 2K^-$$

$$2H_2O \quad \rightleftharpoons \quad 2OH^- \; + \; 2H^-$$

At anode:

$${CH_2COO^- \atop CH_2COO^-} \quad \longrightarrow \quad {CH_2COO \atop CH_2COO} \quad \longrightarrow \quad {CH_2 \atop \| \atop CH_2} \; + \; 2CO_2$$

At cathode:

$$2H^- \; + \; 2e^- \quad \longrightarrow \quad \left[2H\right] \quad \longrightarrow \quad H_2$$

5. **Pyrolysis of quaternary ammonium hydrides (Hofmann Elimination):** When tetra alkyl ammonium hydroxide is heated at 400K, it undergoes elimination reaction known as Hofmann elimination, to form alkene.

$$\left[CH_3CH_2CH_2-\underset{\underset{\overset{|}{C}H_3}{\overset{|}{N}}}{\overset{\overset{CH_3}{|}}{N}}-CH_3\right]OH^- \quad \xrightarrow{heat} \quad CH_3-CH\!=\!CH_2 + H_3C-\underset{}{\overset{\overset{CH_3}{|}}{N}}-CH_3 + H_2O$$

Trimethyl n-propyl   propylene   trimethylamine
ammonium hydroxide

Elimination reactions are the converse of reduction reactions in terms of mechanisms. Two atoms or groups connected with neighboring carbon atoms in the substrate molecule are removed to generate a multiple bond. These responses can take place in one of two ways:

Mechanism of E1 and E2 Reactions

The word E1 denotes a single-molecular elimination process. This mechanism is a two-stage process with just one molecule involved in the rate determining phase. In tertiary alkyl halides, these reactions are relatively prevalent. Consider the reaction of tertiary butyl bromide with alc. KOH. solution, for example.

tert. butyl bromide + KOH (alc.) → 2-methylpropene + KBr + H₂O

Mechanism: It's a one-molecular reaction with the following steps:

Step 1: Carbocation formation: Tertiary butyl bromide is self-ionized to produce tert-butyl carbocation and bromide ion.

tert-butyl bromide → (slow) tert-butyl carbocation

The above stage is a slow one, hence it determines the reaction's pace.

Step 2: Carbocation attack by a nucleophile (OH-): The nucleophile (OH-) removes a proton from one of the methyl groups while simultaneously moving electron pair towards carbon bearing positive charge, producing a double bond.

Because the preceding step is a rapid one, it has no influence on the reaction rate.

Kinetics: Because tertiary butyl bromide self-ionisation is the slowest phase in the reaction, it is the rate controlling step, with the slow step dictating the entire reaction. As a result, the overall rate of the reaction is solely dictated by the substrate concentration and is unaffected by the base concentration.

$$\text{Rate } \alpha \ [(CH_3)_3CBr]$$
$$\text{Rate} = K \ [(CH_3)_3CBr]$$

The reactivity of different alkyl halides towards E1 type reactions is as follows:

Alkyl halide (tertiary > secondary > primary)

The production of a carbocation is the sluggish or rate-determining phase in this scenario. Because tertiary carbocations being the most stable and primary carbocations being least stability, tertiary alkyl halides are found to be the most reactive and primary alkyl halides are the least reactive.

Evidences of the E1 response include:

Since the overall rate of the reaction is dictated only by the concentration of alkyl halides and not by the concentration of base, the elimination process using the E1 mechanism must: • Follow first-order kinetics. As a result, first-order kinetics governs the process.

- They don't have a main hydrogen isotope impact. Because -carbon-hydrogen is lost in the second rapid step, there is no isotope impact in first-order eliminations.
- Because the rate of creation of the carbocation is governed by the first step, the reactivity of the E1 reaction is governed by the rate of formation of the carbocation, which is reliant on the carbocation's stability.

  Stability 3° carbocation against 2° carbocation against 1° carbocation

  Reactivity in E1 reactions is also important:

  3° carbocation against 2° carbocation against 1° carbocation

- Rearrangement occurs with E1 reactions: Because the first (slow) step produces carbocations, they can be rearranged to make more stable carbocations. As a result, the order of carbocation stability is 3°carbocation> 2°carbocation>1°carbocation.

Reaction E1: Orientation E1 reactions follow Saytzeff's rule, which states that the primary result in an elimination reaction is a more branched alkene, which is more stable.

$$CH_3CH_2CH_2CHCH_3 \quad \xrightarrow{\text{alc. KOH}} \quad CH_3CH_2CH\!=\!CHCH_3 \quad + \quad CH_3CH_2CH_2CH\!=\!CH_2$$

$$\overset{|}{\underset{Br}{}}$$

$$\qquad\qquad\qquad\qquad\qquad\qquad 89\% \qquad\qquad\qquad 11\%$$

$$\qquad\qquad\qquad\qquad\qquad \text{Major product} \qquad \text{Minor product}$$

E₂ mechanism: E₂ term implies bimolecular elimination reaction. This mechanism involves a single step bimolecular elimination process. When haloalkanes with β -carbon atom are heated in an alcoholic solution of potassium hydroxide, an alkene is formed.

$$R-\overset{\overset{H}{|}}{\underset{\underset{H}{|}}{C}}\overset{\beta}{}\;\overset{\overset{X}{|}}{\underset{\underset{H}{|}}{C}}\overset{\alpha}{}-H \quad + \quad \underset{(alc)}{KOH} \quad \xrightarrow{\qquad} \quad \underset{alkene}{RHC\!=\!CH_2} \quad + \quad KX \quad + \quad H_2O$$

Haloalkane

$$H-\overset{\overset{H}{|}}{\underset{\underset{H}{|}}{C}}\overset{\beta}{}\;\overset{\overset{Cl}{|}}{\underset{\underset{H}{|}}{C}}\overset{\alpha}{}-H \quad + \quad \underset{(alc)}{KOH} \quad \xrightarrow{\qquad} \quad H_2C\!=\!CH_2 \quad + \quad KCl \quad + H_2O$$

Mechanism: The mechanism involves a single step bimolecular elimination process. The nucleophile OH⁻ removes the proton from β-carbon atom. Simultaneously, the halide ion is lost from the α-carbon and generation of double bond between the two carbons takes place.

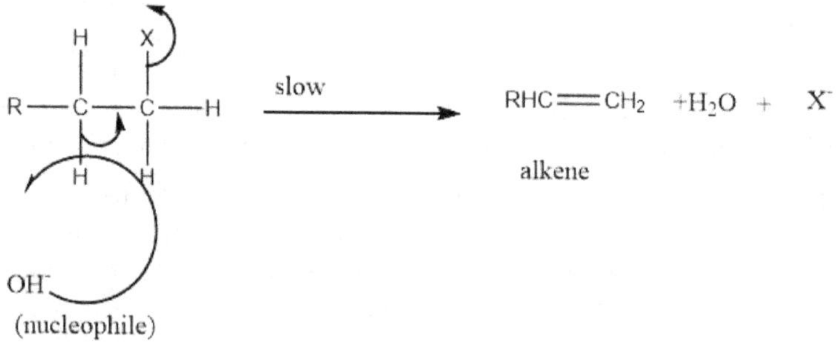

C-H and C-X bonds are concurrently broken in the transition state. The E2 reactions are completed in one step. The base pulls a proton away from carbon, while a halide ion leaves and a double bond is produced. Because the reaction involves a single step and the sluggish rate determining step incorporates both molecules, kinetics is important.

[Alkyl halide] Rate=K [OH-]

The following is the order of reactivity: The reactivity order of different alkyl halides towards E2 type reactions is as follows:

Methyl halide > tertiary > secondary > primary.

The following are examples of evidence for the E2 reaction:

The E2 responses include the following features:

- Second-order kinetics govern E2 reactions.
- E2 reactions do not need rearrangement- Because the rate-determining step comprises a reaction between an alkyl halide molecule and a molecule of base, the resulting kinetics is second order. There are no options for rearranging this single step.

Demonstrate a significant hydrogen isotope effect: Isotope effect refers to a significant change in reaction rate when various isotopes are involved in the reaction.

The fundamental hydrogen isotope effects are shown here, which explains why a protium (H) bond breaks faster than a deuterium (D) one (D). By comparing the rate constants k^H and k^D, the difference in response rate may be calculated.

Consider reaction:

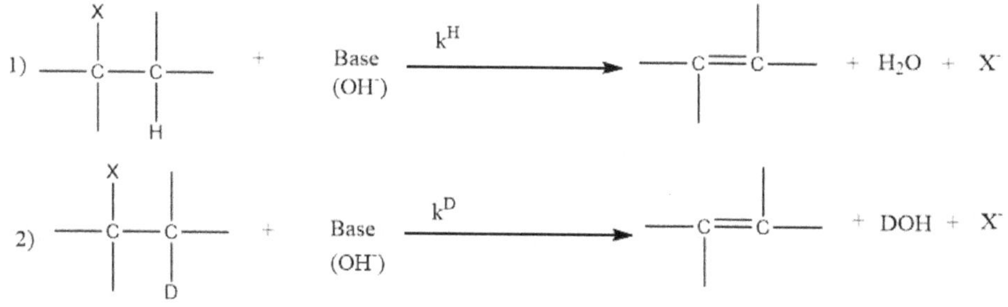

Now $\dfrac{kH}{kD}$ = 5 to 8 (at room temperature)

Thus, above isotope effect shows that breaking of β-carbon -hydrogen bond is rate determining step.

There is a substantial element effect: alkyl halide reactivity follows the order in elimination processes.

$$\text{R-I} > \text{R-Br} > \text{R-Cl} > \text{R-F}$$

Alkyl bromides react 40 to 60 times faster than chlorides, the rate of breaking the carbon-halogen bond influences the overall rate of elimination.

E$_2$ Reaction: Orientation and reactivity (Saytzeff's Rule):

Consider dehydrohalogenation of 2-bromobutane.

$$CH_3CH_2CHCH_3 \xrightarrow{\text{KOH (alc)}} CH_3CH=CHCH_3 + CH_3CH_2CH=CH_2$$
$$\underset{\text{Br}}{|} \qquad\qquad (81\%) \qquad\qquad (19\%)$$

$$CH_3CH_2-\underset{\underset{\text{Br}}{|}}{\overset{\overset{CH_3}{/}}{C}}-CH_3 \xrightarrow{\text{KOH (alc)}} CH_3CH=\underset{\underset{CH_3}{|}}{C}-CH_3 + CH_3CH_2-\underset{\underset{CH_3}{|}}{C}=CH_2$$
$$(71\%) \qquad\qquad (29\%)$$

Chemical Reactions of Alkenes

Russian Chemist Alexander Saytzeff summarized that:

The alkene with the most alkyl groups linked to the doubly linked carbon atoms is the favoured product of dehydrohalogenation.

Ease of formation of alkenes:

$$R_2C=CR_2 > R_2C=CRH > R_2=CH_2 > RCH=CHR > RCH=CH_2 > CH_2=CH_2$$

As a result, according to Saytzeff's rule, the more stable an alkene is, the faster it forms during dehydrohalogenation. The creation of the more stable isomer is referred to as Saytzeff's orientation. The order of reactivity of alkyl halides in E2 dehydrohalogenation is:

The above sequence makes sense since 3° alkyl halides produce highly branched alkenes, which are more stable.

Alkenes have the following chemical properties:

The double bond constitutes of a strong C-C sigma bond and a weak C-C pi bond, bond distinguishes alkenes. The pi-electrons combine to form pi-electron cloud that extends above and below the plane of the carbon atoms that are linked together. As a result, these pi electrons are loosely linked between the two carbon atoms because they are more exposed. Pi-electrons attract electrophiles while repelling nucleophiles due to their negative charge. In other words, alkenes go through electrophilic processes.

1. **Bromine addition:** Bromine reacts with ethylene to generate ethylene dibromide at room temperature.

$$CH_2\!=\!CH_2 \;+\; Br_2 \;\xrightarrow{CCl_4}\; \underset{Br}{\overset{Br}{CH_2\!-\!CH_2}}$$

Ethylene   Ethylenedibromide

Mechanism: The mechanism of addition of bromine to ethylene is electrophilic in nature and consists of the following steps:

Step 1: Formation of cyclic bromonium ion.

$$CH_2\!=\!CH_2 \;+\; Br\text{-}Br \;\xrightarrow{slow}\; \overset{+}{\underset{H_2C-CH_2}{Br}} \;+\; Br^-$$

bromonium ion

Step 2: Formation of trans addition products.

The Br- ion attacks one of the carbon atoms of bromonium ion (from the side opposite to that on which positively charged bromine is present), resulting in the creation of trans addition product.

$$\overset{+}{\underset{H_2C-CH_2}{Br}} \;+\; Br^- \;\xrightarrow{fast}\; \underset{Br}{\overset{Br}{CH_2\!-\!CH_2}}$$

1. Dibromoethane

(Trans product)

2. **Hydrogenation of alkenes:** Alkenes undergo hydrogenation reaction by adding hydrogen, in the presence of finely divided metals to form alkanes. The mechanism of hydrogenation of alkenes follows electrophilic addition

$$\overset{}{\underset{}{C\!=\!C}} \;+\; H_2 \;\xrightarrow{Pt,\ Pd\ or\ Ni}\; \underset{H\quad H}{-C\!-\!C-} \;+\; Heat$$

$$CH_2\!=\!CH_2 \;+\; H_2 \;\xrightarrow{Raney\ Ni}\; CH_3\!-\!CH_3$$

Ethene   Ethane

$$CH_3\!-\!CH\!=\!CH_2 \;+\; H_2 \;\xrightarrow{Raney\ Ni}\; CH_3CH_2CH_3$$

Propene   propane

3. **Addition of halogen halide:** Alkenes readily undergo addition reactions with hydrogen halides to form corresponding alkyl halides.

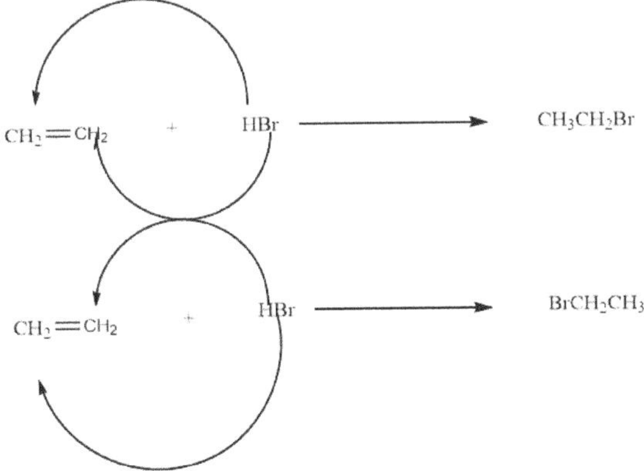

Mechanism: The addition of hydrogen halides to alkenes takes place by two steps electrophilic mechanism:

Mechanism:

Step1: In the first step involves ionisation of halogen acid (HX) to form halogen ion (nucleophile) and proton (electrophile).

Step2: Firstly, the proton attacks the double bond to form carbocation and it further undergoes rearrangement to more stable carbocation as stability order of various carbocations is as:

3°carbocation> 2° carbocation>1° carbocation

Step3: The halogen ion then attacks the carbocation formed to yield alkyl halide.

In case of symmetrical alkenes, the product formed is the same.

On the other hand, in case of unsymmetrical alkenes, there are two alternatives possible For example, consider reaction of propene with HBr.

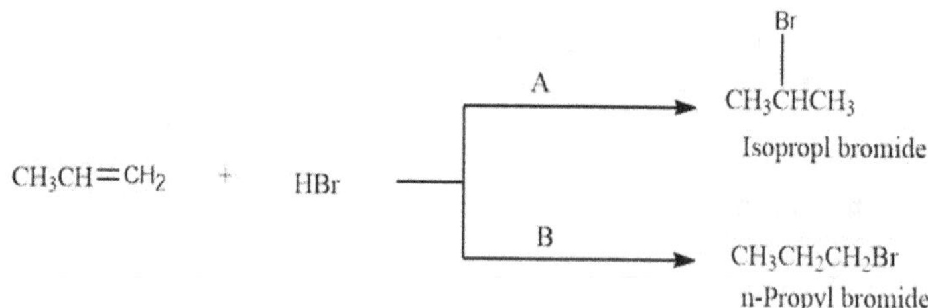

On the reaction of unsymmetrical alkenes with halogen acids, two products are feasible, but only one is obtained as the preferable product, which is in accordance with Markovnikov's Rule.

In 1869, Russian scientist Markovnikov studied a large number of similar addition reactions and established an empirical rule that became known as Markovnikov's rule after his name. The following is the text of the regulation:

The positive component of an unsymmetrical reagent clings to the doubly bonded carbon with the most hydrogen atoms when it interacts with an unsymmetrical alkene. Or

When unsymmetrical reagents like HX, H_2O, HOX, and others are added to unsymmetrical alkenes, the negative component of the contributing molecule is directed to the carbon atom of the double bond with the fewest hydrogen atoms.

As a result, we may claim that the product created by route A is the primary product in the aforementioned reaction.

Markovnikov's Rule: A Theoretical Explanation

Because the addition reaction halogen halides with alkenes follows electrophilic addition mechanism. The attack of proton to propene is first step in the addition reaction of HBr. There are two ways to add something. A 2° carbocation (I) is created when the proton contributes to the double bond's terminal carbon atom; a 1° carbocation (II) is created when the proton contributes to the intermediate carbon atom.

Carbocation (I) is formed more frequently than carbocation (II) because a 2° carbocation (I) is more stable. The Br-ion then nucleophilically attacks this carbocation, generating 2-bromopropane as the major product.

As a result, Markovnikov's addition takes place via a more stable intermediate carbocation.

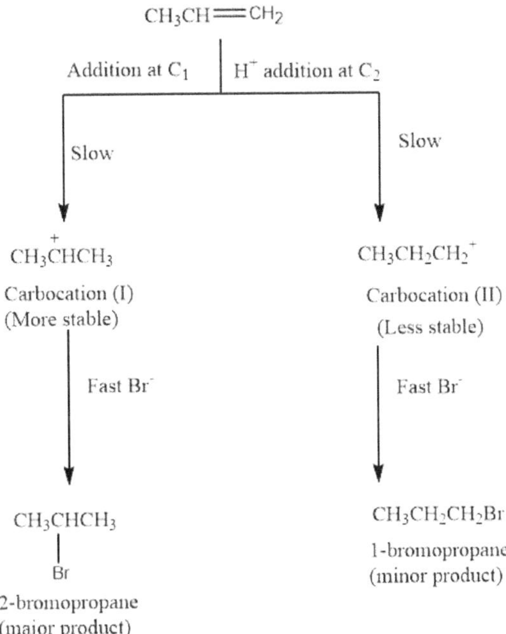

4. **Hydrogen halide addition in the presence of peroxide (Kharasch effect)-** Propylene displays the addition reaction with HBr in the presence of peroxide to generate 1-bromopropane which is different from the one expected in the absence of peroxide.

$$CH_3CH=CH_2 \; + \; HBr \xrightarrow{\text{Peroxide}} CH_3CH_2CH_2$$
$$|$$
$$Br$$

1-bromopropane

Because the result is opposite of what Markovnikov's Rule predicts, it's known as Anti Markovnikov's Rule.

Mechanism: It is based on the free radical process and includes the following phases.:

Step1- Chain initiating step: Organic peroxide undergoes homolysis to form free radical.

$$R\text{-}O\text{-}O\text{-}R \xrightarrow{\text{Homolysis}} 2R\text{-}O$$

Alkoxy free radical

$$R\text{-}O \; + \; H\text{-}Br \longrightarrow R\text{-}OH \; + \; Br$$

Bromine free radical

Step2- Chain propagating step: The bromine radical produced attacks propene molecule so as to produce more stable free radical.

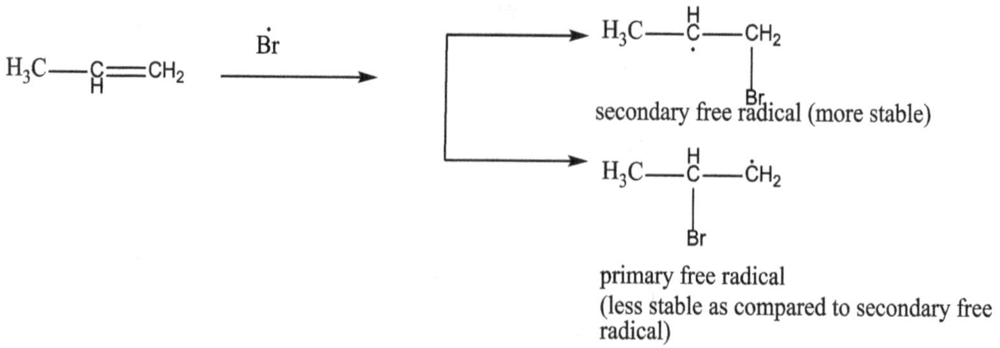

Since secondary free radical is more stable, it will be preferably formed. The secondary free radical then reacts with HBr to form 1-bromopropane and bromine free radical.

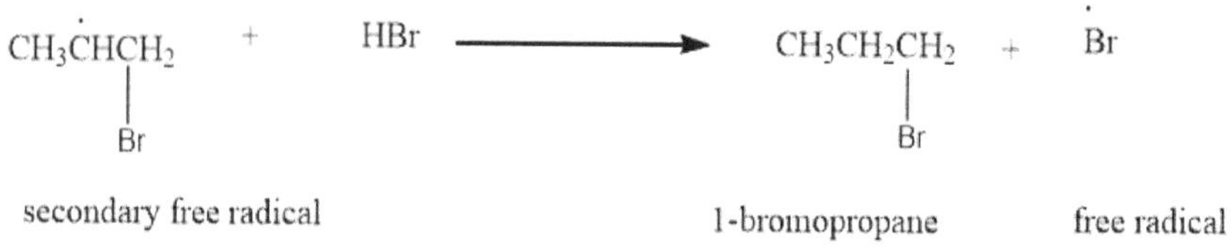

This bromine radical continues the chain by repeating the chain propagating step.

Step 3: Chain terminating step: At the end, the reaction stops by coupling the free radicals formed in the reaction.

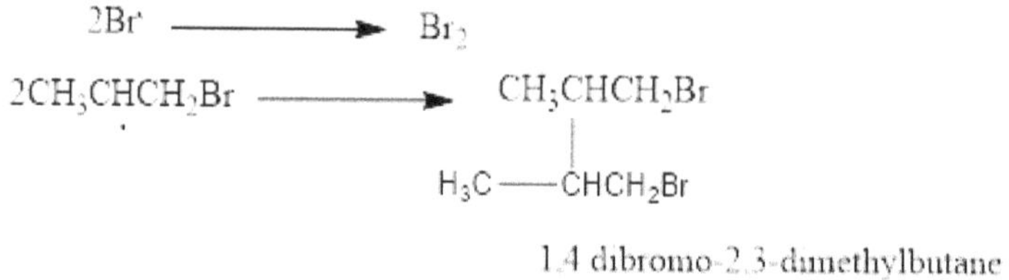

5. **Formation of halohydrin**: The reaction between alkenes and bromine or chlorine in the presence of water results in the formation of halohydrins. In general, reaction can be represented as:

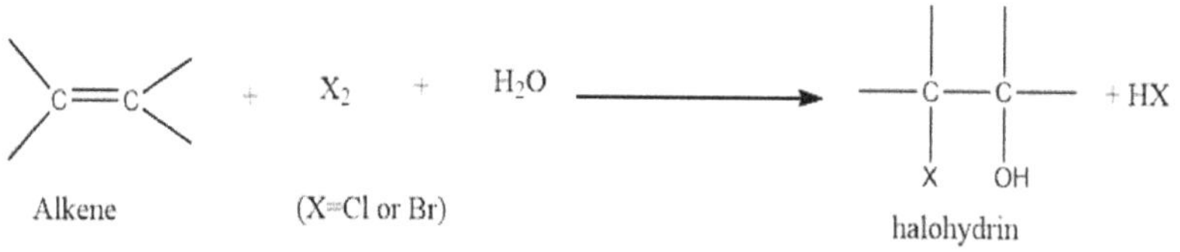

For example,

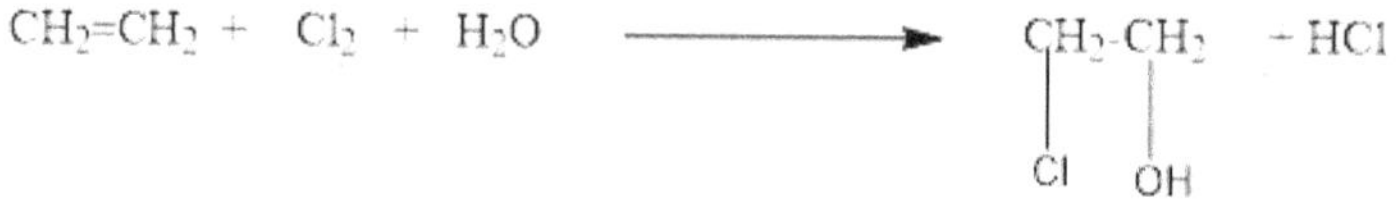

6. **Addition of sulphuric acid-** Cold conc. sulphuric acid (H_2SO_4) reacts with alkenes to give alkyl hydrogen. sulphates.

$$\text{Alkene} \quad + \quad H_2SO_4 \quad \longrightarrow \quad \text{Alkyl hydrogen sulphate} \ (OSO_2OH)$$

For example,

$$CH_2{=}CH_2 \quad + \quad H_2SO_4 \quad \longrightarrow \quad CH_3{-}CH_2OSO_2H$$

ethylene   Ethyl hydrogen sulphate

7. **Addition of alkanes**: **Alkylation**: Alkenes add on alkanes in the presence of suitable acidic catalysts to form larger alkanes. The addition is alkylation and generally employed for the commercial manufacture of alkanes such as 2,2,3-trimethylpentane which is used as aviation fuel.

$$\text{Alkene} \quad + \quad R{-}H \quad \xrightarrow{\ H^+\ } \quad \text{Higher alkane} \ (H, R)$$

For example,

$$H_3C{-}\underset{CH_3}{C}{=}CH_2 \ + \ H_3C{-}\underset{CH_3}{CH}{-}CH_3 \quad \xrightarrow{\ H_2SO_4\ } \quad CH_3{-}\underset{H}{\overset{CH_3}{C}}{-}CH_2{-}\underset{CH_3}{\overset{CH_3}{C}}{-}CH_3$$

Isobutylene   isobutane   2.2-trimethylpentane

8. **Addition of alkenes: Polymerization**: Under suitable conditions molecules of an alkene join together to form large molecules called polymers. The reaction is known as polymerization reaction.

Polymerization of alkenes is also known as addition polymerization or vinyl polymerization:

Formation of polyethylene or polyethene ($-CH_2CH_2)_n$ takes place by heating pure ethylene at 463-483K temperature under 1500 atmospheric pressure in the presence of traces of oxygen.

Similarly, Polypropene can be prepared by passing propylene through n-hexane containing triethyl aluminium at 373K under 10 atmospheric pressure.

$$nCH_2=CH_2 \xrightarrow[\text{traces of oxygen}]{463\text{-}483 \text{ K,1500 atm}} (-CH_2-CH_2-)_n$$

$$nCH_3-CH=CH_2 \xrightarrow[\text{10atm. 373K}]{(C_2H_5)_3Al} (-\underset{\underset{CH_3}{|}}{CH}-CH_2-)_n$$

propylene

propylene

9. **Hydroboration-oxidation of alkenes**: When alkenes are treated with diborane $(BH_3)_2$, alkenes undergo hydroboration to form alkyl boranes. The alkyl boranes get oxidised by hydrogen peroxide in alkaline solution to form alcohols.

$$H_2C=CH_2 \quad + \quad (BH_3)_2 \longrightarrow CH_3CH_2BH_2 \xrightarrow{CH_2=CH_2} (CH_3CH_2)_2BH$$

Ethylene

ethylborane

Diethylborane

$$CH_2=CH_2 \downarrow$$

$$3CH_3CH_2OH \quad + \quad H_3BO_3 \xleftarrow{OH^-} 3H_2O_2 + (CH_3CH_2)_3B$$

ethyl alcohol

triethylborane

Hydroboration-oxidation is also a regioselective reaction and the alcohol obtained is such as if anti-Markownikoff addition of water to alkenes had taken place. Thus this method can be used for the preparation of alcohols which cannot be prepared by other methods of hydration of alkenes.

10. **Ozonolysis:** Ozonolysis is a process in which ozone is added to a double bond to form an ozonide, which is then disintegrated into lower pieces containing aldehydes and/or ketones. Ozonides are combustible compounds that are impossible to separate. When heated with zinc and water, ozonides cleave at the double bond's seat.

Oxidation with hot KMnO₄: When alkenes react with hold concentrated $KMnO_4$, alkenes split at the double bond to form ketones and acid.

$$CH_3-\underset{\underset{CH_3}{|}}{C}=CH-CH_3 \xrightarrow[\text{hot KMnO}_4]{[O]} CH_3-\underset{\underset{CH_3}{|}}{C}=O \quad + \quad CH_3COOH$$

Acetone

Acetic acid

Dienes

Dienes are bifunctional chemicals with two double bonds between carbon and carbon in the molecule. C_nH_{2n-2} is the general formula that describes them. Alkadienes is another name for them. Dienes are classified into three groups based on the locations of their double bonds:

(i) **Isolated or non-conjugated dienes**: Isolated dienes have more than one single bond between their double bonds.

As an example,

$$CH_2=CH-CH=CH_2 \qquad\qquad CH_2=CH-CH=CH-CH_3$$

Buta-1,3-diene   Penta-1,3-diene

(ii) **Conjugated or Alternating Dienes:** Conjugated dienes have a single bond between two double bonds. For example,

$$CH_2=CH-CH=CH_2 \qquad\qquad CH_2=CH-CH=CH-CH_3$$

Buta-1,3-diene   Penta-1,3-diene

(iii) **Cumulated dienes:** Cumulated dienes or allenes are dienes with two double bonds connected to the same carbon atom.

For example,

$$H_2C=C=CH_2 \qquad\qquad H_2C=C=\underset{H}{C}-CH_2CH_3$$

Propa-1,2-diene or allene   Penta-1,2-diene

Conjugated dienes are the most important of all the three classes of dienes.

Structure of conjugated dienes and non-conjugated dienes:

Let us consider conjugated diene as buta-1,3-diene. Each of the four carbon of buta-1,3 diene uses three sp^2 hybrid orbitals for the formation of σ bonds and an unhybridized p-orbital for the formation of π-bonds. Each C-H bond is sp^2-s sigma bond and each C-C bond is sp^2-sp^2 sigma bond. There are four pure unhybridized p-orbitals, one on each carbon atom. The p-orbital of C_1 overlaps the p-orbital of C_2 and the p-orbital of C_3 and C_4 overlap sidewise, leading to structure (ii) In short, there is an overlapping of p-orbitals of C_1 with C_2, C_2 with C_3 and C_3 with C_4, leading to structure (iii). Therefore, all the four p-orbitals result in the formation of π-molecular orbital which covers all the four carbon atoms, leading to structure (iv).

In other words, we can say that the π-electron cloud is not localised between any of the two carbon atoms but instead spreads over and is delocalised over all the four carbon atoms. The delocalisation is responsible for the lesser energy content and stability of conjugated dienes.

On the other hand, the non-conjugated dienes such as penta-1,4 diene ($CH_2=CH-CH_2-CH=CH_2$), there is formation of two π-bonds. These are formed by the sidewise overlap of the unhybridized orbitals belonging to C_1 and C_2 carbon atoms as well as C_4 and C_5 carbon atoms. Since the carbon atom C_3 is sp^3 hybridised and has no unhybridised orbital, this carbon is not involved in any type of overlapping. Hence, there is no delocalisation possible in case of non-conjugated dienes (isolated dienes). Thus, conjugated dienes are more stable than non-conjugated dienes.

Thus, a conjugated diene such as buta-1,3-diene is a resonance hybrid of the following structures:

$$CH_2=CH-CH=CH_2$$
(i)

$$CH_2-CH=CH-CH_2$$
(ii)

$$\overset{+}{CH_2}=CH-CH_2-\overset{-}{\underset{..}{CH}}$$
(iii)

$$\overset{+}{CH_2}-CH=CH-\overset{-}{\underset{..}{CH_2}}$$
(iv)

Structure (ii) has got a formal bond between C_1 and C_4 (dotted line) because of the pairing of the electrons on C_1 and C_4 atoms which have opposite spins. The effective bond between these atoms cannot be formed because the distance between them is quite large. There is a separation of charges in structure (iii) and (iv). The structure (i) is quite stable because it had more number of effective bonds and at the same tome it does not involve separation of charges. Thus actual structure of buta-1,3 diene is a hybrid of structures (i), (ii), (iii) and (iv) in which structure (i) has maximum contribution.

The C-C single bonds in 1,3-butadiene are shorter (1.48A°) than normal carbon-carbon single bonds whereas they are longer than normal isolated carbon-carbon double bonds.

The delocalisation of π-electron charge because of resonance leads to increase the stability of buta-1,3-diene (conjugated diene), the resonance energy being 14.6kJmol^{-1}.

On the other hand, isolated diene, penta-1,4-diene is written in two resonating structures, out of which only structure (v) makes the contribution while structure (vi) due to charge separation had very less contribution.

$$CH_2=CH-CH_2-CH=CH_2 \longleftrightarrow \overset{+}{CH_2}-\underset{..}{CH}-CH_2-CH=CH_2$$

(v)   (vi)

Since the number of contributing structures for penta1,4-diene is less than the buta-1,3-diene, therefore, a conjugated diene is more stable than the isolated diene.

Preparation of Dienes

1. **By the dehydrohalogenation of 1,3 dichlorobutanes**: Isoprene can be prepared by the dehydrohalogenation of 1,3-dichloro-3-methyl butane with alcoholic KOH.

$$CH_3-\underset{\underset{CH_3}{|}}{\overset{\overset{Cl}{|}}{C}}-CH_2-CH_2-Cl \xrightarrow[\text{heat}]{KOH(alc)} CH_2=\underset{\underset{}{}}{\overset{\overset{CH_3}{|}}{C}}-CH=CH_2$$

1,3-DIchloro-3-methylbutane   3-methyl but-1,3-diene

2. **By dehydration of butane-1,4-diol-** When a butane-1,4-doil is heated with conc. H_2SO_4, buta-1,3-diene is formed.

$$CH_2-CH_2-CH_2-CH_2 \xrightarrow[\text{heat}]{\text{conc.}H_2SO_4} H_2C=CH-CH=CH_2 \quad + \quad 2H_2O$$

Butane-1,4-diol   Buta-1,3-diene

3. **By pyrolysis of cycloalkenes (retro-Diels-Alder reaction)-** Buta-1,3-diene is synthesised by passing cyclohexene vapours through a heated nichrome (Ni-Cr-Fe) alloy.

Cyclohexene   Buta-1,3-diene   ethylene

Chemical Reactions of Dienes

1. **Electrophilic addition of conjugated dienes i.e., 1,4-addition and 1,2 addition:**

When 1,3 butadiene is treated with bromine, not only is the predicted result 3,4-bromo-1-butene produced, but also 1,4 dibromo 2-butene is obtained.

Mechanism: The mechanism of electrophilic addition reaction of dienes is as follows:

Step1: HBr ionises to give a proton (electrophile) and a bromide ion (nucleophile)

$$HBr \longrightarrow H^+ + Br^-$$

Step2: Now proton attacks a double bond according to Markovnikov's Rule so as to give most stable carbonium ion.

$$H^+ + CH_2=CH-CH=CH_2 \longrightarrow$$

$$CH_3\text{-}\overset{+}{C}H\text{-}CH=CH_2 \quad (A)$$

$$CH_3\text{-}CH=CH\text{-}\overset{+}{C}H_2 \quad (B)$$

Step3: Bromide ion Br^- combines with either cation (A) or (B) to form the final product. When Br^- combines with (A), one gets 1,2 addition product whereas if Br^- combines with (B), 1,4 addition product is obtained. Hence, a mixture of product is obtained.

$$\xrightarrow{\text{Br}_2}$$

$$\underset{\underset{\text{Br}}{|}\ \underset{\text{Br}}{|}}{\text{CH}_2\text{-CH-CH=CH}_2} \quad \text{(1,2 addition)}$$

$$+$$

$$\underset{\underset{\text{Br}}{|}\ \ \ \ \ \ \underset{\text{Br}}{|}}{\text{CH}_2\text{-CH=CH-CH}_2}$$

(1,4-addition)

$$\text{CH}_2\text{=CH-CH=CH}_2 \xrightarrow{\text{HCl}} \underset{\underset{\text{H}}{|}\ \underset{\text{Cl}}{|}}{\text{CH}_2\text{-CH-CH=CH}_2} \quad \text{(1,2 addition)}$$

$$+$$

$$\underset{\underset{\text{H}}{|}\ \ \ \ \ \ \underset{\text{Cl}}{|}}{\text{CH}_2\text{-CH=CH-CH}_2}$$

(1,4 addition)

$$\xrightarrow{\text{H}_2} \underset{\underset{\text{H}}{|}\ \underset{\text{H}}{|}}{\text{CH}_2\text{-CH-CH=CH}_2} \quad \text{(1,2 addition)}$$

$$+$$

$$\text{CH}_3\text{-CH=CH-CH}_3$$

(1,4 addition)

$$\overset{+}{\text{CH}_3\text{-CH-CH=CH}_2} \ + \ \text{Br}^- \longrightarrow \underset{\underset{\text{Br}}{|}}{\text{CH}_3\text{-CH-CH=CH}_2}$$

(A)   3-Bromo-1-butene

$$\overset{+}{\text{CH}_3\text{-CH=CH-CH}_2} \ + \ \text{Br}^- \longrightarrow \text{CH}_3\text{-CH=CH-CH}_2\text{Br}$$

(B)   1-bromo-2-butene

Carbocation (B) is produced in higher amounts than carbocation (A) because it is more stable. Because it is an allylic cation, it is resonance stabilized, yielding 1-bromo-2-butene (1,4 addition product) as the major product, while carbocation (A) is produced in less quantities, yielding 3-bromo-1-butene (1,2 addition product) as the minor result.

1,2 -Addition: vs. 1,4 (Kinetically and thermodynamically regulated processes) Rate versus Equilibrium:

When HBr is added to 1,3-butadiene, it creates both the 1,2-addition and 1,4-addition products; the amounts in which they are formed are heavily determined by the reaction temperature. The reaction creates a mixture that contains 20% of the 1,4-addition product and 80% of the 1,2-addition product at -80°C. The reaction yields a mixture of compositions at a higher temperature (40°C), with 80 percent 1,4-addition product and 20 percent 1,2-addition product.

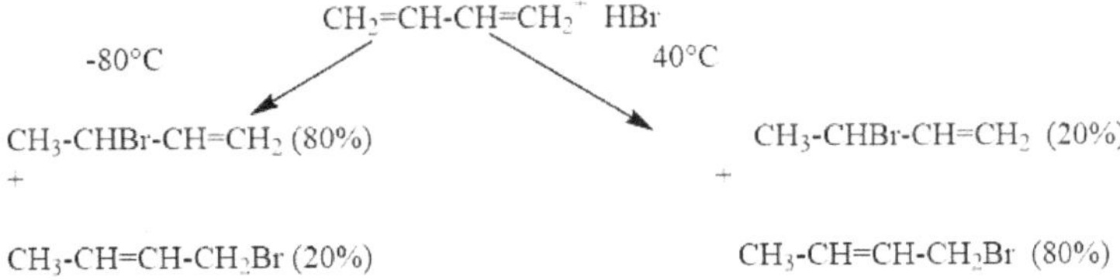

At -80°C, more 1,2-addition product is created than 1,4-addition product, showing that 1,2-addition product is created quicker. The originally created products are gradually transformed into the equilibrium mixture as the reaction temperature rises.

The proportions of products successfully separated from low-temperature addition are governed by the rates of addition, whereas the proportions of products actually separated from high-temperature addition are dictated by the equilibrium between the two isomers.

Furthermore, it is seen that the carbocations initially produced react to generate the 1,2-addition product more faster than the 1,4-addition product, implying that the energy of activation leading to the 1,2-addition product must be less than that leading to the 1,4-addition product. As a result, it is depicted as a smaller slope that leads from the cation to the 1,2-addition product. The 1,4-addition product, on the other hand, is more stable, and its valley is located at a lower level than the 1,2-addition product.

Potential energy changes during progress of reactions: 1,2-addition product vs 1,4-addition product:

Ionisation of bromides entails ascending potential hills back to this carbocation. However, there is a higher hill separating the cation from the 1,4-addition product than there is between the 1,2-addition product; as a result, the 1,4-addition product will ionise more slowly than the 1,2-addition product. When the rates of the opposing reactions are equal, equilibrium is attained. The 1,2-addition product forms quickly but ionises slowly, yet the 1,4-addition product persists once formed. The more stable1,4-addition product predominates at temperatures high enough to attain equilibrium and allow for significantly quick ionisation.

2. **Diel's Alder reaction**: 1,3 -butadiene combines with an alkene or alkyne to form cyclic compound. In this reaction alkene or alkyne act as dienophile and reacts with diene to form product of Diel's alder reaction known as adduct. The net reaction involves formation of two new σ bonds and one new π bond at the expense of three original π-bonds. It involves intermolecular cyclisation reaction (cycloaddition reaction) between a 4π- electron system (a diene) and a 2π- electron system (an alkene or alkyne). It is also called (4+2) cycloaddition reaction. The alkene (a 2π system) called dienophile adds on to diene to form Diels Alder adduct. The simplest example of this reaction is addition of ethene to but-1,3-diene to give cyclohexane.

Buta-1.3-diene   ethene(dienophile)   cyclohexene

Mechanism: The 1,4-addition of an alkene molecule to a conjugated diene is the mechanism. The reaction takes place in a single step, with the conjugated diene system's C-1 and C-4 attaching to the dienophile's doubly-bonded carbons. As a result, at the expense of two diene and dienophile links, two new bonds are formed. bonds.

Buta-1,3-diene   Ethene   Cyclohexene

Diel's alder reaction can be used to the preparation of cyclic compounds which were otherwise difficult to prepare.

MCQs

1. Which of the following reaction is used for the preparation of alkane?
   (a) Corey-House synthesis
   (b) Williamson synthesis
   (c) Friedal craft's reaction
   (d) None of these

2. Among the option which one is not reactive towards sulphuric acid?
   (a) Alkene
   (b) Alkyne
   (c) Alcohol
   (d) Alkane

3. Why is halogenation of alkanes considered as chain reaction?
   (a) It occurs quickly
   (b) Each step generates the reactive intermediate for the further steps
   (c) No intermediates is formed
   (d) The reaction leads to long chain halogenated alkanes

4. The chlorination of alkane gives:
   (a) Free radical substitution reaction
   (b) Nucleophilic addition

   (c) Electrophilic substitution

   (d) Electrophilic addition

5. Formation of chlorine radical in chlorination of alkanes is called

   (a) Propagation   (b) Activation

   (c) Deactivation   (d) Initiation

6. Chlorination as compared to bromination proceeds at:

   (a) Faster rate   (b) Equal rates

   (c) Slower rate   (c) Depends on types of alkane

7. The methods not used for the preparation of alkanes:

   (a) Hydrogenation of alkenes or alkynes

   (b) Reduction of alkyl halides

   (c) Halogen exchange reaction

   (d) Frankland methods

8. Kolbe's electrolysis of sodium butyrate ($CH_3CH_2CH_2COO^-Na^+$) gives:

   (a) C_8H_{16} (b) C_6H_{14}

   (c) C_8H_{18} (d) C_6H_{12}

9. Paraffins are:

   (a) Alkene   (b) Alkyne

   (c) Alkane   (d) Alkyl halides

10. The hybridization of alkenes is

   (a) sp^3 (b) sp^2

   (c) sp (d) None of the above

Answers for MCQs

1. (a)	2. (d)	3. (b)	4. (a)	5. (d)
6. (a)	7. (c)	8. (c)	9. (c)	10. (b)

Short Answer Questions

1. What are alkanes? What do you know about their chemical reactivity?

2. What do you mean by paraffins? Write their uses.

3. Write short note on sp^3 hybridisation of alkanes.

4. Arrange the structural isomers of pentane in decreasing order of their boiling point.

5. An alkane with molecular weight 72 formed only one monochloro-substitution product. Suggest structure for the alkane.

6. How many sigma bonds are there in molecule of ethane and ethene?

7. Why does methane not react with Cl_2 in the dark?

8. Explain why alkanes are inert.

9. Give limitations of Wurtz reaction.

10. Write structures of all possible chloroethanes produced during free radical chlorination of ethane.

11. Arrange the following sets of alkenes in decreasing order of stability:

    (i) 1-Butene, cis-2-butene, isobutylene and trans-2-butene

    (ii) 1-Pentane, 2-methyl-2-butene, cis-2-pentene, trans-2-pentene.

12. Predict the products formed when 2-butene reacts with diazomethane in the presence of light.

13. What do you mean by Saytzeff's rule. Explain with the help of example.

14. Write down the order of reactivity of various carbocations.

15. An alkene on ozonolysis yields acetone and formaldehyde. Write its structure and IUPAC names.

16. What do you mean by Markownikoff's rule? Give example.

17. Write the structures of alkenes which gives a mixture of propanone and methanal on ozonolysis.

18. Predict the product obtained on treatment of propene with HI in the presence of peroxide.

19. What id the major product formed when 2-bromobutane is treated with alc. KOH?

20. What is Diel's Alder reaction?

21. Explain why buta-1,3diene is more stable than penta-1,3diene.

22. What do you mean by Baeyer's reagent used to check unsaturation in alkenes and alkynes.

23. Explain sp^2 hybridisation in alkenes.

24. Write short note on Saytzeff's orientation.

Long Answer Questions

1. How does stability of free radicals play a role in the halogenation of alkanes?

2. Write short notes on:

    (i) Corey-House reaction

    (ii) Wurtz reaction

3. Though I-I bond is very weak, but the iodination of alkanes does not take place readily. Explain.

4. Write short note on reactivity and selectivity of alkanes in the halogenation of alkanes.

5. Discuss Kolbe's reaction and decarboxylation of carboxylic acids for the formation of alkanes.

6. Discuss the mechanism of chlorination of methane and give three evidences in support of the above mechanism.

7. Calculate the % age of expected isomers during monobromination of n-butane. The relative rates of substitution per 3°, 2° and 1° hydrogen are 1600: 82: 1.

8. What is Wurtz reaction? Discuss its mechanism. Is this method suitable for the synthesis of unsymmetrical alkanes? If not, why?

9. Convert:

   (i) Ethane into butane by Corey-House reaction.

   (ii) Propanoic acid to ethane.

10. Dehydration of alcohols to form alkenes is generally carried out by heating with conc. H_2SO_4.

    (a) Why cannot we use a base in place of H_2SO_4?

    (b) Why HNO_3 or HCl cannot be used in place of H_2SO_4?

11. What do you understand by 1,2-hydride shift? Explain with suitable examples from dehydration of alcohols.

12. What do you mean by Ozonolysis reaction. Explain with mechanism.

13. Discuss the mechanism of addition of bromine to 1,3-butadiene.

14. Explain why 1,3-butadiene undergoes 1,2- and 1,4-addition reaction.

15. What are different classes of diene? Which of these represents the most stable dienes? Explain.

16. Give structures and names of products expected from the reaction of each of the following with 1,3-butadiene:

    (i) 1mole of H_2 (ii) 2 moles of HI   (iii) 1 mole of Br_2

    (iv) 2 moles of bromine   (v) 1mole of HCl   (vi) 2 moles of HCl.

17. Give the mechanism of 1,2 and 1,4 addition of buta-1,3 diene. What is the effect of temperature on the addition of Br_2 to buta-1,3 diene.

18. Discuss the effect of temperature upon the formation of products during reaction of HBr with 1,3-butadiene.

19. Give any three methods for the preparation of diene.

20. Explain allylic substitution in alkenes.

21. What is Peroxide effect?

22. Give detailed mechanism for E1 and E2 elimination. Enlist important difference between two mechanisms.

23. Explain Markownikoff's and anti- Markownikoff's addition of hydrogen halide to unsymmetric alkenes.

24. The relative reactivity of 1°, 2°, 3° hydrogen's towards chlorination is 1 : 3.8 : 5. Calculate the percentages of all monochlorinated products obtained from 2-methylbutane.

25. Why do alkenes prefer to undergo electrophilic addition reaction while arenes prefer electrophilic substitution reactions? Explain.

26. Alkynes on reduction with sodium in liquid ammonia form trans alkenes. Will the butene thus formed on reduction of 2-butyne show the geometrical isomerism?

Alkyl Halides and Alcohols

Alkyl Halides

Alkyl halides or mono haloalkanes or simply haloalkanes or simply haloalkanes are the halogen derivatives of alkanes. The usual formula is CnH_{2n+1}-X, where n=1,2,3,..., and X is any halogen atom such as F,Cl, Br, or I. Alkyl halides are formed when one or more hydrogen atoms in an alkane are replaced with appropriate halogen atoms. For example,

CH_3Br	CH_3CH_2Cl	$CH_3CH_2CH_2I$
Bromoethane	Chloroethane	Iodopropane
Br-CH_2CH_2-Br	CH_3CHCl_2	$CHCl_3$
1,2-dibromoethane	1,1-dichloroethane	Trichloromethane
$Cl_2CHCH_2CH_2Cl$	$CHCl_3$	$_0CCl_4$
1,1,3-Trichloropropane	Trichloromethane	Tetrachloromethane

Classification of alkyl halides:

Depending on whether the X atom is connected to a primary, secondary, or tertiary carbon, alkyl halides can be classed as primary (1°), secondary (2°), or tertiary (3°).

Example:

Primary alkyl halides:

CH_3CH_2Cl	$CH_3CH_2CH_2Br$
Chloroethane	1-Bromopropane
(Isopropyl bromide)	(n-Propyl bromide)

Secondary alkyl halides:

$CH_3CHBrCH_3$ $CH_3CHClCH_2CH_3$

2-Bromopropane	2-Chlorobutane
(Isopropyl bromide)	(sec-Butyl chloride)

Tertiary alkyl halides:

$C(CH_3)_3Cl$	$CH_3C(CH_3)BrCH_2CH_2CH_3$
2-Chloro-2methylpropane	2-Bromo-2methylpentane
(tert-Butyl chloride)	(tert-hexylbromide)

Preparations of Alkyl Halides

Alkyl halides can be made in a variety of ways, as shown below:

1. **By halogenation of alkanes**: A complex combination of isomeric mono- and poly-haloalkanes is generated by free radical halogenation of alkanes (usually bromination and chlorination) in the presence of UV light or at high temperature (400°C)

$$CH_4 \xrightarrow[\text{UV light}]{Cl_2} CH_3Cl + CH_2Cl_2 + CHCl_3 + CCl_4$$

Methane

$$CH_3CH_2CH_2CH_3 \xrightarrow[\text{or heat}]{Cl_2/\text{UV light}} ClCH_2CH_2CH_2CH_3 + CH_3CHCH_2CH_3$$

Butane

Isomeric monochloro compounds +

Isomeric monodichloro compounds

Hence, halogenation of alkane is not suitable for the halogenation of pure haloalkanes in the laboratory because a mixture of haloalkanes are obtained which are difficult to separate into individual products due to little difference in the boiling points of different products.

2. **Addition of halogen halide:** Alkenes are easily converted to alkyl halides by reacting with hydrogen halides (HCl, HBr, or HI).

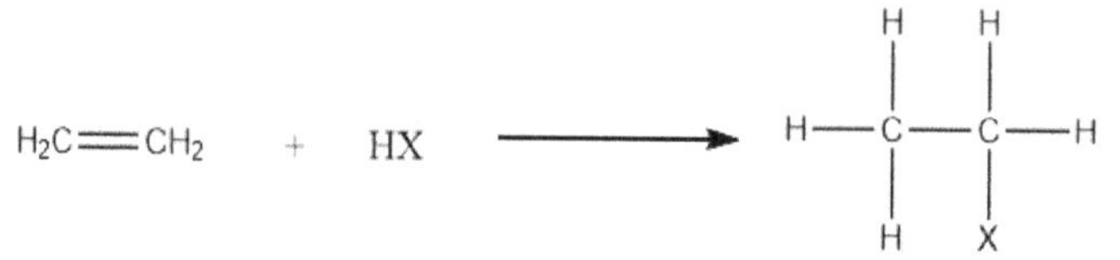

$$H_2C{=}CH_2 + HX \longrightarrow$$

Ethylene   ethyl iodide

Mechanism: The addition of hydrogen halides to alkenes takes place by two steps electrophilic mechanism:

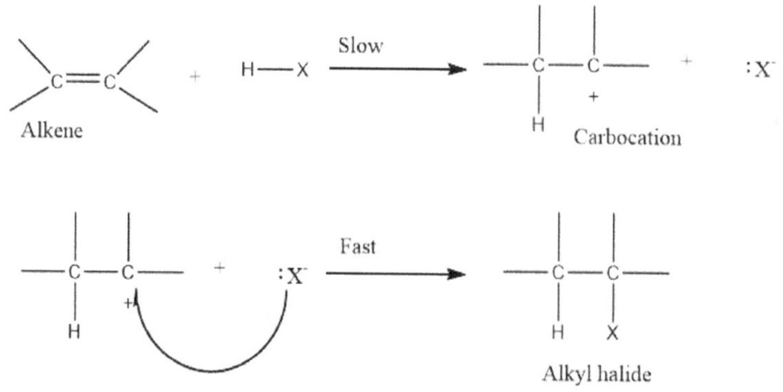

Alkene   +   H—X $\xrightarrow{\text{Slow}}$ Carbocation   +   :X⁻

   +   :X⁻ $\xrightarrow{\text{Fast}}$ Alkyl halide

Mechanism:

Step1: The first step involves ionisation of halogen acid (HX) to form halogen ion (nucleophile) and proton (electrophile).

Step2: Firstly, the proton attacks the double bond to form carbocation and it further undergoes rearrangement to more stable carbocation as stability order of various carbocations is as:

3°carbocation> 2° carbocation>1° carbocation

Step3: The halogen ion then attacks the carbocation formed to yield alkyl halide.

In the case of symmetrical alkenes, the product generated is same regardless of how H-Br attaches to the alkene.

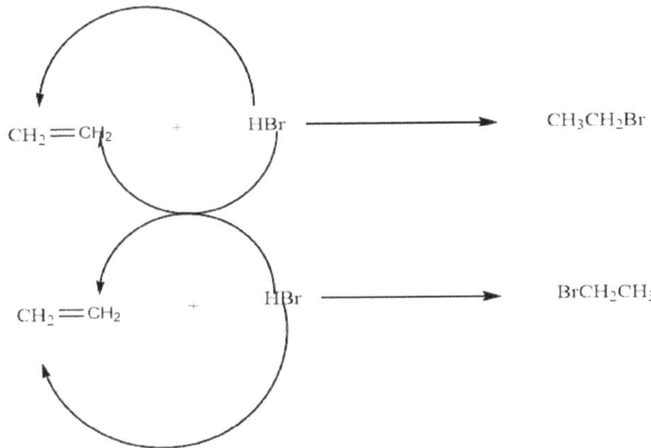

On the other hand, in case of unsymmetrical alkenes, there are two alternatives possible

For example, consider reaction of propene with HBr

$CH_3CH=CH_2$ + HBr → A → $CH_3\overset{\displaystyle Br}{\overset{|}{C}}HCH_3$ Isopropl bromide

→ B → $CH_3CH_2CH_2Br$ n-Propyl bromide

On the reaction of unsymmetrical alkenes with halogen acids, two products are feasible, but only one is produced as the main product, which is in accordance with Markovnikov's Rule. In 1869, Markovnikov, a Russian chemist, researched a large number of similar addition reactions and proposed an empirical rule that is now known as Markovnikov's rule. The following is the rule: When an asymmetrical reagent reacts with an asymmetrical alkene, the positive half of the reagent attaches to the doubly bonded carbon that has the most hydrogen atoms.   Or

When unsymmetrical reagents like HX, H_2O, HOX, and others are added to unsymmetrical alkenes, the negative component of the adding molecule goes to the carbon atom of the double bond that has the least amount of hydrogen atoms. Hence, we can say that in above reaction product formed by pathway A is the major product.

Theoretical explanation of Markovnikov's Rule:

Because the electrophilic addition reaction of halogen halides to alkenes. As a result, the initial step in the addition of HBr to propene is to add a proton. The addition might take two forms. A 2° carbocation (I) is generated when the proton adds to the double bond's terminal carbon atom, whereas a 1° carbocation (II) is generated when the proton adds to the intermediate carbon atom.

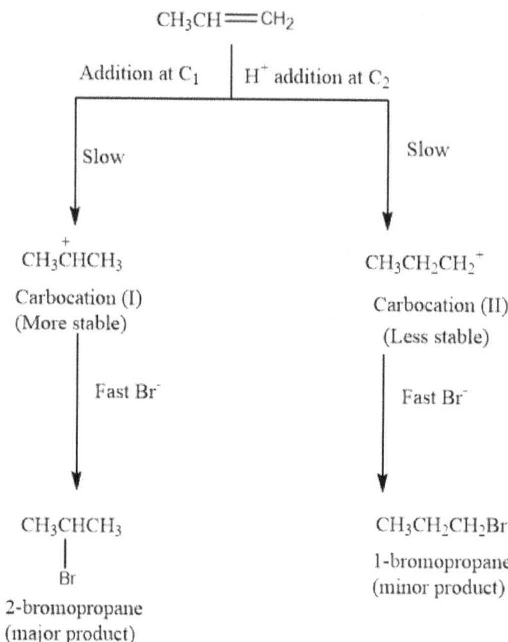

Because a 2° carbocation (I) is more stable than a 1° carbocation (II), carbocation (I) is generated more frequently. The Br-ion then attacks this carbocation nucleophilically, generating 2-bromopropane as the main result. As a result, Markovnikov's addition is accomplished via a more stable carbocation intermediate.

Addition of hydrogen halide in the presence of peroxide (Kharasch effect)-

In the presence of peroxide, propylene interacts with HBr to generate 1-bromopropane.

$$CH_3CH = CH_2 \ + \ HBr \xrightarrow{\text{Peroxide}} CH_3CH_2CH_2 - Br$$

1-bromopropane

Because the result is the polar opposite of what Markovnikov's Rule predicts, it's also known as Anti Markovnikov's Rule.

Mechanism: Its proceeds with free radical mechanism and consists of the following steps:

Step1- Chain initiating step: Homolysis transforms organic peroxide into a free radical.

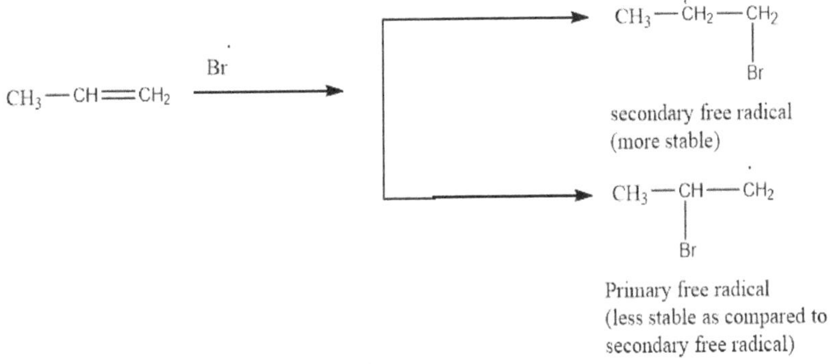

Step2- Chain propagating step: The bromine radical then adds to propene molecule in such a way that the more stable free radical is produced.

As the secondary free radical is more stable, it will be preferably formed. The secondary free radical then reacts with HBr to form 1-bromopropane and bromine free radical.

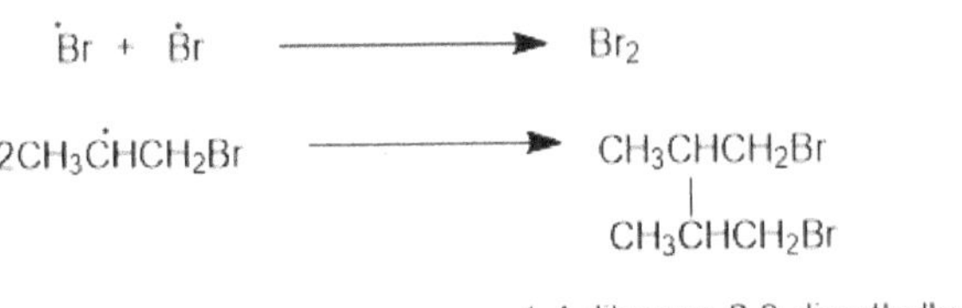

This bromine radical continues the chain by repeating the chain propagating step.

Step3: Chain terminating step: At the end, the reaction stops by coupling the free radicals formed in the reaction.

3. **By treating alcohols with suitable reagents**: The halogen atom is substituted for the -OH group of alcohol in the preparation of haloalkanes. The following strategies can be used to accomplish this:

(i)   Hydrochloric acid gas is passed through a suitable alcohol in the presence of anhydrous zinc chloride to produce alkyl chlorides. Grove's procedure is the name given to this procedure.

$$CH_3CH_2OH + HCl\,(g) \xrightarrow{\text{Anhydrous ZnCl}_2} CH_3CH_2Cl + H_2O$$

Ethanol   Chloroethane

$$CH_3\underset{\underset{\displaystyle OH}{|}}{CH}CH_3 + HCl\,(g) \xrightarrow{\text{Anhydrous ZnCl}_2} CH_3\underset{\underset{\displaystyle Cl}{|}}{CH}CH_3 + H_2O$$

Propan-2-ol   2-chloropropane
(Isopropyl alcohol)

In the aforementioned reaction, $ZnCl_2$ acts as a catalyst by assisting in the cleavage of the C-O bond. Because it is a Lewis acid, it coordinates with the oxygen atom of alcohols, weakening the C-O bond and resulting in carbocation.

(i) Bromoalkanes or alkyl bromides can be made by refluxing a suitable alcohol with continual boiling HBr (48%) in the presence of a little amount of conc.H_2SO_4.

$$CH_3CH_2\text{-}OH + HBr \xrightarrow[\text{Reflux}]{H_2SO_4} CH_3CH_2Br + H_2O$$

                                                           Bromoethane

(ii) **By action of Phosphorus halides**: By reacting a certain alcohol with phosphorus trichloride or phosphorus pentachloride, chloroalkanes or alkyl chlorides are created.

$$3CH_3CH(OH)CH_3 + PCl_3 \longrightarrow 3CH_3CH(Cl)CH_3 + H_3PO_3$$

Propan-2-ol   Phosphorus   2-chloropropane   Phosphorus acid
                      trichloride

$$CH_3CH_2OH + PCl_5 \longrightarrow CH_3CH_2Cl + POCl_3 \;+\; HCl$$

Ethanol   Phosphorus   Chloroethane   Phosphorus
                pentachloride   oxychloride

(iii) **By using thionyl chloride**: Alcohols can also be made into alkyl chloride by refluxing them with thionyl chloride in the presence of pyridine. Darzen's response is another name for this response.

$$CH_3CH_2OH \quad SOCl_2 \xrightarrow{\text{pyridine}} CH_3CH_2Cl + SO_2 + HCl$$

                                                     chloroethane

Alkyl chlorides are best prepared by this method as the by products are in gaseous form and hence escape readily from the reaction mixture. Pyridine is used in the reaction as it consumes HCl formed as the product and hence helps to proceed the reaction in the forward direction.

4. Finkelstein reaction or halogen exchange reaction: An alkyl iodide can be made by combining sodium iodide with an alkyl chloride or bromide in a methanol or acetone solution.

$$CH_3CH_2Cl + NaI \xrightarrow[\text{heat}]{\text{Acetone}} CH_3CH_2I + NaCl$$

Chloroethane · · · · · · · · · · · · · Iodoethane

$$CH_3CH_2Br + NaI \xrightarrow[\text{heat}]{\text{Acetone}} CH_3CH_2I + NaCl$$

Bromoethane · · · · · · · · · · · · · Iodoethane

5. **Hunsdiecker reaction**: In a carbon tetrachloride solution, a silver salt of carboxylic acid is decomposed by chlorine or bromine to generate an alkyl or aryl halide with one carbon atom fewer than the original acid.

$$RCOOAg + Br_2 \xrightarrow[\text{reflux, 350K}]{CCl_4} R\text{-}Br + AgBr + CO_2$$

Silver salt of
carboxylic acid

$$CH_3COOAg + Br_2 \xrightarrow[\text{reflux, 350K}]{CCl_4} CH_3Br + AgBr + CO_2$$

Silver acetate · · · · · · · · · · · · · Bromomethane

Chemical Reactions of Alkyl Halides

Because the halogen atom in haloalkanes is more electronegative than the carbon atom, alkyl halides are very reactive. As a result, the C-X bond's shared pair of electrons is polarised, shifting toward the more electronegative halogen atom. As a result, the carbon atom gains a little positive charge (+), whereas the halogen atom gains a little negative charge (-). Alkyl halides are highly reactive compounds due to the existence of tiny positive and negative charges on carbon and halogen atoms. They go through a number of substitution, elimination, and reduction processes.

(A) Substitution reactions: Because the halogen atom has a higher electronegativity than the carbon atom, the carbon-halogen bond in alkyl halides is polar. As a result, the carbon atom has a partial positive charge (+) and is a favourable target for nucleophiles. The most prevalent alkyl halide reactions are nucleophilic substitution reactions. They can be written as:

Nucleophile · · · · · · · Alkyl halide · · · · · · · Substitution product · · · · · · · Leaving group

Nucleophilic substitution can proceed by two mechanisms:

S_N^1 **Mechanism**: Unimolecular nucleophilic substitution (S_N^1) is a kind of nucleophilic substitution that occurs in a single molecule. The reaction occurs in two phases in this mechanism, and the rate of the reaction is determined solely by the concentration of alkyl halide and is unaffected by the concentration of nucleophile.

As a result, the kinetics of SN1 reactions are first order. Consider tertiary butyl bromide hydrolysis with the hydroxide ion.

$$H_3C-\underset{\underset{CH_3}{|}}{\overset{\overset{CH_3}{|}}{C}}-Br \;+\; \underset{(aq)}{KOH} \longrightarrow H_3C-\underset{\underset{CH_3}{|}}{\overset{\overset{CH_3}{|}}{C}}-OH \;+\; KBr$$

tert. Butylbromide   tert. Butylalcohol

Mechanism: It is unimolecular reaction and consists of the following steps:

Step1: Formation of carbocation: The alkyl halide ionizes to give a planar carbocation and bromide ion. The carbocation is planar because the central positively charge carbon atom is sp^2 hybridized.

$$H_3C-\underset{\underset{CH_3}{|}}{\overset{\overset{CH_3}{|}}{C}}-Br \underset{\text{rate determining step}}{\overset{\text{slow}}{\rightleftharpoons}} H_3C-\underset{\underset{CH_3}{|}}{\overset{\overset{CH_3}{|}}{C}}^{+} \;+\; Br^-$$

t-Butyl bromide   t-Butyl carbocation

Because this phase is sluggish, it determines the reaction's pace.

Step2: Attack of nucleophile on carbocation: The carbocation formed in Step1 readily combines with nucleophile (OH⁻) to form tertiary butyl alcohol.

$$H_3C-\underset{\underset{CH_3}{|}}{\overset{\overset{CH_3}{|}}{C}}^{+} \;+\; OH^- \overset{\text{Fast}}{\longrightarrow} H_3C-\underset{\underset{CH_3}{|}}{\overset{\overset{CH_3}{|}}{C}}-OH$$

tert-Butyl carbocation   tert-Butylalcohol

This phase is quick, therefore it has no bearing on the reaction's speed.

Rearrangement in SN^1 reactions:

Carbocations formed in the first step may:

   (a) combine with a nucleophile

   (b) rearrange to a more stable carbocation.

As stability order of various carbocations is as:

3°carbocation> 2° carbocation>1° carbocation.

In the first phase of the SN1 process, carbocations are rearranged to generate more stable carbocations. Such a rearrangement occurs when a 1,2-alkyl shift of hydrogen or alkyl may generate a more stable carbocation. The nucleophile and the newly created carbocation combine to generate the substitution product.

For example, Consider the n-propyl cation, which may be converted to the more stable isopropyl cation by shifting hydrogen.

Primary carbocation

Secondary carbocation
(more stable)

Primary carbocation undergoes rearrangement to form secondary carbocation (more stable)

In case of the 3,3 dimethyl-2-butyl cation, a methyl shift takes place to yield a tertiary cation. This type of shift is known as methyl shift.

A secondary carbocation

Tertiary carbocation

Secondary carbocation undergoes rearrangment to form more stable tertiary carbocation

As in all previous carbocation reactions, the electron-deficient carbon atom obtains a pair of electrons in rearrangement, but this time at the price of a surrounding carbon atom that can better tolerate the positive charge.

Kinetics: Because tert-butyl bromide ionisation is the slowest stage in the reaction, the pace of the reaction is solely determined by the concentration of tert-butyl bromide.

The response rate is calculated as follows:

Rate of the reaction α [(CH$_3$)$_3$C-Br]

Rate of the reaction = k [(CH$_3$)$_3$C-Br], where k is constant of proportionality

Stereochemistry: $S_N{}^1$ reactions occur through carbocation intermediate which is sp^2 hybridised and planar in character. The three positively charged carbon substituents in a plane are 120° apart, with the empty p-orbital perpendicular to the plane. Now, as can be seen from the image of the carbocation, the nucleophile, OH$^-$, may approach the carbocation from both sides with equal ease.

When the nucleophile attacks the carbocation on the front side, the product has the same configuration as the reactant because the nucleophile occupies the same location in the product as the leaving group did in the reactant. If the nucleophile approaches from the rear, however, an alcohol is formed, but with the conformation inverted. Thus, racemic mixture of product is produced.

(Enantiomers)

Order of reactivity towards S_N^1 reaction is:

Tertiary > Secondary > Primary

This is because the production of carbocation is a rate-determining step in the SN1 reaction. The tertiary carbocation is more stable and so easier to produce, implying that ionisation of the tertiary alkyl halide is advantageous. In the case of secondary alkyl halides, the secondary carbocation is less stable, but in the case of primary alkyl halides, the primary carbocation is the least stable and hence hardest to generate.

As a result, the reactivity of alkyl halides towards the SN1 reaction is in the following order:

Tertiary > Secondary > Primary.

S_N^2 **mechanism**: The abbreviation SN2 stands for Substitution nucleophilic bimolecular reactions are single-step reactions in which the rate of reaction is determined by the concentration of alkyl halide and nucleophile.

For example, consider the action of nucleophile on primary alkyl halide.

$$R\text{-}CH_2\text{-}X \;\; + \;\; Nu^- \longrightarrow R\text{-}CH_2\text{-}Nu \;\; + \;\; X^-$$

Primary alkyl halide

$$\text{Rate } \alpha \; [R\text{-}CH_2X][Nu^-]$$

Thus, S_N^2 reactions show second order kinetics. Let us consider the hydrolysis of methyl bromide (primary alkyl halide) by the hydrolysis of methyl bromide (primary alkyl halide) by the hydroxyl ions ion aqueous solution.

$$CH_3Br \; + \;\; OH\text{-} \longrightarrow CH_3OH \; + \;\; Br\text{-}$$

Methyl bromide

Mechanism: The nucleophile attack and the ejection of the alkyl halide happen at the same time in this process. From the rear side, the base's OH- ion assaults the methyl bromide molecule. It can strike from the same side as the negatively polarised bromine, but it will be repulsed. The reactants travel through a transition state where the C-OH bond is half-formed and the C-X bond is half-broken on their path to the products.

Bromomethane   slow step   Transition state   Methanol (inversion of configuration)   + Br

Since S_N^2 mechanism proceeds in single step, rearrangement is not possible in S_N^2 mechanism.

Kinetics: Because the production of the transition state is a long process involving the collision of methyl bromide with the hydroxyl ion, the pace of the reaction is influenced by the concentrations of both methyl bromide and hydroxide ion.

$$\text{Rate } \alpha \; [\text{Methyl bromide}] \; [OH^-]$$

$$\text{Rate} = K \; [\text{Methyl bromide}] \; [OH^-]$$

Where K is constant of proportionality

Stereochemistry: The entering nucleophile hits the alkyl halide molecule from the backside in SN2 reactions. As a result, the molecule's conformation is reversed. The product generated as a result of the SN2 process has an inverted conformation in the case of optically active alkyl halides. The hydrolysis of (-) 2-bromooctane with aqueous sodium hydroxide solution, for example, uses the SN2 process to produce (+) octan-2-ol. The configuration of (+) octan-2-ol is the polar opposite of (-) 2-bromooctane.

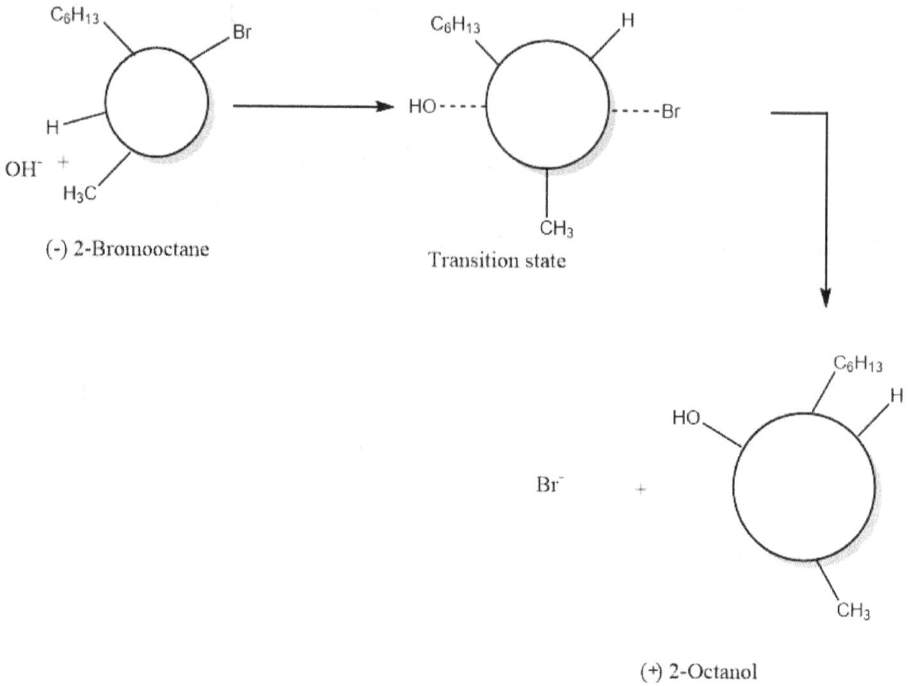

C6H13 · Br · H · OH⁻ + · H3C

(-) 2-Bromooctane

C6H13 · H · HO---- · ----Br · CH3

Transition state

C6H13 · H · HO · Br⁻ + · CH3

(+) 2-Octanol

Thus, In the case of optically active substances, SN2 reactions are invariably followed by full configuration inversion.

Order of reactivity of various alkyl halides towards S_N^2 reactions is:

Primary > Secondary > Tertiary

This is because the development of a transition state is a rate-determining step in the SN2 reaction. The nucleophilic assault on the backside of the alkyl halide catalyses the SN2 reaction. Like the wind inverting an umbrella, this back-side assault inverts the carbon atom tetrahedron. In the case of primary alkyl halides, this form of assault is rather simple. The carbon atom is bonded to halogen and then coupled to three alkyl groups in a tertiary alkyl halide. The approaching nucleophile is hampered by these bulky alkyl groups. Stearic hindrance is the name given to this sort of impediment. Secondary alkyl halides, on the other hand, have fewer alkyl groups than tertiary alkyl halides, and hence encounter less stearic hindrance. Because primary alkyl halides have the least stearic hindrance, they may easily undertake SN2 reactions. As a result, the reactivity of alkyl halides towards SN2 type reactions is in the following order:

Primary > Secondary > Tertiary.

Factors effecting S_N^1 and S_N^2 mechanism:

The various factors which effect S_N^1 and S_N^2 mechanism are given as follows:

(i) **Structure of alkyl halide**: The SN2 mechanism is favoured by primary alkyl halides. Tertiary alkyl halides, on the other hand, favour the SN1 mechanism. Secondary alkyl halides are equally suited to each of these processes.

(ii) Nature of nucleophile: Powerful nucleophiles such as negative nucleophile (RO^- and OH^-) favour S_N2 mechanism where the substitution is completed in a single step. The weak nucleophiles (H_2O and ROH) favour S_N1 mechanism where the substitution is completed in two steps.

(iii) Nature of the solvent: Ionization of alkyl halides is aided by polar solvents such as alcohol and water. As a result, polar solvents like benzene and carbon tetrachloride favour the SN1 process because a carbocation intermediate is produced during this mechanism, whereas non-polar solvents like benzene and carbon tetrachloride favour the S_N2 process. **(iv) Concentration of nucleophile**: Because the rate of reaction in the S_N2 mechanism follows second order kinetics and is dependent on the concentration of nucleophile, the rate of reaction increases as the concentration of nucleophile rises. The S_N1 mechanism, on the other hand, follows first-order kinetics, and the rate of reaction is independent of nucleophile concentration.

Differences between S_N^1 mechanism and S_N^2 mechanism:

S_N1 mechanism	S_N2 mechanism
1. It is governed by first-order kinetics.	1. It is governed by second-order kinetics.
2. It is completed in two steps.	2. It is completed in one step.
3. Carbocations are formed as intermediates	3. The reaction is completed in a single step.
4. The nucleophile can attack from the back side as well as from the front side and hence racemic mixture of product is obtained.	4. Nucleophile can attack only from the back side and inverted product is obtained.
5. Racemic mixture of product is obtained.	5. The arrangement is completely inverted.
6. The order of reactivity of alkyl halides is: Tertiary > Secondary > Primary	6. The order of reactivity of alkyl halides is: Primary > Secondary > Tertiary
7. It is accompanied by rearrangement so that most stable carbocation is obtained.	7. No rearrangement is possible since the reaction is completed in a single step.
8. Favoured by weak nucleophiles such as alcohols and water	8. Favoured by strong nucleophiles such as alkoxide.
9. Reactions are favoured by polar solvents.	9. Usually favoured by non-polar solvents.
10. The rate of the reaction is unaffected by the concentration of nucleophile.	10. As the concentration of nucleophile rises, so does the rate of reaction.

Some of the substitution reactions of alkyl halide as given as follows:

1. **Reaction with alkoxide**: On heating alkyl halides with sodium alkoxides, alkyl halides are converted into ethers.

$$R\text{-}X + RO^-Na^+ \xrightarrow{\text{heat}} R\text{-}O\text{-}R + NaX$$

Alkyl halide   Sodium alkoxide   ether

$$C_2H_5\text{-}Br + CH_3O^-Na^+ \xrightarrow{\text{heat}} CH_3\text{-}O\text{-}C_2H_5 + NaBr$$

Bromoethane   Sodium methoxide   Methoxyethane

$$C_2H_5\text{-}Br + C_2H_5O^-Na^+ \xrightarrow{\text{heat}} C_2H_5\text{-}O\text{-}C_2H_5 + NaBr$$

Bromoethane   Sodium ethoxide   Ethoxymethane

This reaction is known as Williamson's synthesis for ethers.

2. **Formation of alcohols:** Alkyl halides form corresponding alcohols on boiling with aqueous alkali solution or with most silver oxide.

$$R\text{-}X + K^+OH^-(aq) \xrightarrow{\text{boil}} R\text{-}OH + KX$$

Alkyl halide   Alcohol

$$C_2H_5\text{-}Br + K^+OH^-(aq) \xrightarrow{\text{boil}} C_2H_5\text{-}OH + KBr$$

Bromoethane   Ethanol

$$C_2H_5\text{-}I + Ag^+OH^- \xrightarrow{\text{boil}} C_2H_5OH + AgI$$

Iodomethane moist silver   Ethanol
oxide

3. **Reaction with cyanides**: Alkyl halides react with alcoholic solution of potassium cyanide to give substituted alkanenitriles (alkyl cyanides).

$$R\text{-}X + K^+CN^-(alc) \xrightarrow{\text{heat}} R\text{-}CN + KX$$

Alkanenitrile

$$CH_3\text{-}I + K^+CN^- \xrightarrow{\text{heat}} CH_3CN + KI$$

Iodomethane   (alc)   methyl cyanide

$$C_2H_5Cl + K^+CN^- \xrightarrow{\text{heat}} C_2H_5\,CN + KCl$$

Chloromethane   (alc)   ethyl cyanide

4. **Formation of esters**: Alkyl halides are converted into esters on heating with silver salts of acids.

$$R\text{-}X + RCOO^-Ag^+ \longrightarrow R\text{-}COOR + AgX$$
Alkyl halide   silver salt   Ester

$$CH_3\text{-}Br + CH_3COO^-Ag^- \longrightarrow CH_3COOCH_3 + AgBr$$
Methyl bromide   Silver acetate   Methyl acetate

$$C_2H_5\text{-}Cl + CH_3COO^-Ag^+ \longrightarrow CH_3COOC_2H_5 + AgCl$$
Ethyl chloride   Silver acetate   Ethyl acetate

5. **Formation of nitroalkanes**: Alkyl halides in aqueous alcoholic solution react with silver nitrite upon heating to form nitroalkanes.

$$R\text{-}X + Ag\text{-}O\text{-}N{=}O \longrightarrow RNO_2 + AgX$$
Alkyl halide Silver nitrite   Nitroalkane

$$C_2H_5\text{-}Br + Ag\text{-}O\text{-}N{=}O \longrightarrow C_2H_5NO_2 + AgBr$$
Bromoethane   Silver nitrite   Nitroethane

6. **Formation of alkyl nitrites**: Alkyl nitrites are formed when alkyl halides combine with sodium or potassium nitrite.

$$R\text{-}X + K^-O^-\text{-}N{=}O \longrightarrow R\text{-}O\text{-}N{=}O + KX$$
Alkyl halide Potassium   Alkyl nitrite
              nitrite

$$C_2H_5Br + K^+O^-\text{-}N{=}O \longrightarrow C_2H_5\text{-}O\text{-}N{=}O + KBr$$
Bromoethane   Potassium   Ethyl nitrite
              nitrite

7. **Reaction with ammonia**: A combination of primary, secondary, tertiary amines, and quaternary ammonium salt is generated when alkyl halides are heated with an alcoholic ammonia solution in a sealed tube at 373K.

$$C_2H_5\text{-}Br + H\text{-}NH_2 \xrightarrow[\text{heat}]{C_2H_5OH} C_2H_5\,NH_2 + HBr$$

Bromoethane   Ethylamine

$$C_2H_5\text{-}Br + H\text{-}NHC_2H_5 \xrightarrow[\text{heat}]{C_2H_5OH} C_2H_5\text{-}NH\text{-}C_2H_5 + HBr$$

Diethylamine

$$C_2H_5\text{-}Br + H\text{-}N(C_2H_5)_2 \xrightarrow[\text{heat}]{C_2H_5OH} (C_2H_5)_3N + HBr$$

Triethylamine

$$(C_2H_5)_3N + C_2H_5\text{-}Br \xrightarrow[\text{heat}]{C_2H_5OH} (C_2H_5)_4N^+Br^-$$

Tetraethylammonium bromide

8. **Formation of higher alkynes**: When alkyl halides are treated with sodium alkynides, higher alkynes are formed.

$$R\text{-}X + R\text{—}C\equiv C^-Na^+ \longrightarrow R\text{—}C\equiv C\text{—}R + NaX$$

Alkyl halide   Sodium alkyanide   Higher alkyne

$$CH_3\text{-}Br + H\text{—}C\equiv C^-Na^+ \longrightarrow H\text{—}C\equiv C\text{—}CH_3 + NaBr$$

Bromoethane   Sodium acetylide   Propyne

9. **Formation of thioalcohols**: Thioalcohols are formed by heating alkyl halides in an aqueous alcoholic solution of sodium or potassium hydrosulphide.

$$R\text{-}X + Na^+S^-H \xrightarrow[\text{heat}]{C_2H_5OH/H_2O} R\text{-}SH + NaX$$

Alkyl halide   Thioalcohol

$$C_2H_5Br + Na^+S^-H \xrightarrow[\text{heat}]{C_2H_5OH/H_2O} C_2H_5SH + NaBr$$

Bromoethane   Ethanethiol

10. **Reduction of alkyl halides**: Alkanes are formed from haloalkanes by following reagents:

(a) **Using nascent hydrogen**: It is liberated by treating Zn or Sn with HCl or Zn-Cu and alcohol.

$$Zn + 2HCl \longrightarrow ZnCl_2 + 2[H]$$

Nascent

$$C_2H_5I + 2[H] \longrightarrow C_2H_6 + HI$$

Iodomethane   Ethane

(b) By using H_2 in the presence of catalyst (catalytic reduction): It takes place in the presence of Pt, Ni, or Pd metals.

$$C_2H_5Br + H_2 \xrightarrow{\text{Ni}} C_2H_6 + HBr$$

Bromoethane   Ethane

(c) By using HI in the presence of red phosphorus: The reaction is carried out at about 420K.

$$C_2H_5I + H\text{-}I \xrightarrow[\text{420K}]{\text{Red P}} C_2H_6 + I_2$$

Ethyl iodide   Ethane

Elimination Reactions

(A) Elimination reactions/ dehydrohalogenation reactions: Alkenes are produced when haloalkanes are heated in an alcoholic solution of potassium hydroxide. The reaction continues with the removal of a hydrogen halide molecule. The hydrogen in the hydrogen halide that is removed comes from the - carbon (i.e. the carbon atom adjacent to the one carrying the halogen) while the halogen atom comes from the - carbon (i.e. the carbon atom carrying halogen atom).

Ethyl bromide   ethene

n-propyl bromide   Propylene

This reaction is an example of 1,2 elimination since it involves the removal of a halogen atom and a hydrogen atom from a beta-carbon next to the one losing the halogen, thus the name.

Mechanism: The mechanism involves a single step bimolecular elimination process. The nucleophilic OH⁻ removes the proton from β-carbon atom. Simultaneously, the halide ion is lost from the α-carbon and a C=C bond is formed.

The cleavage of C-H and C-X bonds requires energy and this comes from:

- The formation of bond between the abstracted proton (H^+) and hydroxide ion (OH^-).
- Formation of π- bond which supplies about $284 kJmol^{-1}$ of energy.
- The energy of solvation of the halide ion.

Orientation/ Regioselectivity:

(i)   In some cases, dehydrohalogenation yields single alkene.

$$CH_3CH_2CH_2CH_2Br \xrightarrow{\text{alc. KOH}} CH_3CH_2CH{=}CH_2 \; + \; KBr \; + \; H_2O$$

1-bromobutane   But-1-ene

$$CH_3CH_2CH{-}CH_3 \; (Br) \xrightarrow[\text{heat}]{\text{KOH (alc)}}$$

$CH_3{-}CH{=}CH{-}CH_3$
But-2-ene (80%)

$CH_3{-}CH_2{-}CH{=}CH_2$
But-1-ene (20%)

2-Bromobutane

The formation of but-2-ene as the primary product follows Saytzeff's rule, which stipulates that the dehydrohalogenation process produces a more strongly substituted alkene with fewer hydrogen atoms on the doubly linked carbon atoms.

(B) Reactions with metals:

(i)   **Reaction with sodium metal-** Higher alkanes are formed when alkyl halides are reacted with metallic sodium in the presence of dry ether. This is known as the Wurtz response.

$$\text{R-X} + 2Na + \text{X-R} \xrightarrow{\text{dry ether}} \text{R-R} + 2NaI$$

Alkyl halide   Alkane

$$CH_3I + 2Na + ICH_3 \xrightarrow{\text{dry ether}} CH_3\text{-}CH_3 + 2NaI$$

Methyl iodide   Ethane

(ii)   **Reaction with lithium**: In the presence of dry ether, alkyl halides react with lithium to generate alkyl lithium.

$$R\text{-}X \;+\; 2Li \xrightarrow{\text{Dry ether}} R\text{-}Li \;+\; LiBr$$
Alkyl lithium

$$C_2H_5Br \;+\; 2Li \xrightarrow{\text{Dry ether}} C_2H_5Li \;+\; LiBr$$
Bromoethane   Ethyl lithium

(iii)   **Action with magnesium:**

$$R\text{-}X \;+\; Ag\text{-}O\text{-}N{=}O \longrightarrow RNO_2 \;+\; AgX$$
Alkyl halide   Silver nitrite   Nitroalkane

$$C_2H_5\text{-}Br \;+\; Ag\text{-}O\text{-}N{=}O \longrightarrow C_2H_5NO_2 \;+\; AgBr$$
Bromoethane   Silver nitrite   Nitroethane

(iv)   **Reaction with copper compound or Corey- House reaction-** Both symmetrical and unsymmetrical alkanes may be produced in good yields using the Corey-House reaction. Alkyl halide is treated with lithium dialkyl copper to produce alkanes in this process.

$$R'\text{-}X \;+\; R_2CuLi \longrightarrow R\text{-}R' \;+\; RCu \;+\; Lix$$
Alkyl halide   lithium dialkyl copper   alkane

For example,

$$CH_3CH_2CH_2Br \;+\; (CH_3)_2CuLi \longrightarrow CH_3CH_2CH_3 \;+\; CH_3Cu \;+\; LiBr$$
n-Butyl bromide   lithium dimethyl copper   n-propane   Methyl copper

Uses of Alkyl Halides

Trichloroethylene (TCE):

Cl   Cl
  C=C
Cl   H

Molecular formula: C_2HCl_3

Uses:

(i)   It is utilised in anaesthesia because of its analgesic effects, which are effective even at low doses. Because of its toxicity, the US Food and Drug Administration (FDA) prohibited these applications of trichloroethylene in 1977, as well as its usage in cosmetics and drugs.

Trichloroethylene exposure, both acute (short-term) and chronic (long-term), can disrupt the human central nervous system (CNS), causing symptoms such as dizziness, headaches, confusion, euphoria, facial numbness, and weakness.

(ii) Trichloroethylene is used in the metal finishing, automotive, and aerospace sectors as a solvent to remove grease from metal components and as a degreasing solvent. TCE is a useful solvent for degreasing soft metals like aluminium and for cleaning steel prior to galvanising. TCE has a number of characteristics that make it a good degreasing agent, including high solvency, low flammability, non-corrosiveness, and high stability. TCE is also a low-cost cleaner that cleans completely and rapidly.

(a) TCE may also be used to extract vegetable oils from plants like coconut and palm.

(b) TCE is also utilised in the manufacturing of 100 percent ethanol to remove residual water.

(c) TCE is used as a feedstock to make hydrofluorocarbon refrigerants and other chlorinated end products, such as flame retardant compounds, in high purity grades. TCE is also utilised in the production of polyvinyl chloride as a molecular weight control agent (PVC).

Tetrachloroethylene

Molecular formula: $Cl_2C=CCl_2$

Uses:
1. Tetrachloroethylene is an anthelmintic used chiefly in the treatment of hookworm infestation.
2. Paint removers, water repellents, silicone lubricants, spot removers, adhesives, wood cleaners, and a wide range of hobbyist items include it. However, in the United States, the use of tetrachloroethylene for dry cleaning has been phased out, and any new usage have been prohibited since 2008.
3. Tetrachloroethylene is employed as grain fumigant.
4. In the automotive and other metal working sectors, it's also used to degrease metal parts.
5. Tetrachloroethylene is used in dry cleaning, textile processing, as a chemical intermediary, and in metal-cleaning processes for vapour degreasing.
6. Moreover, it is used as excellent solvent for organic material in pharmaceutical industries.

Chloroform

Molecular formula: $CHCl_3$

Uses:

1. Chloroform has been commonly used as an anaesthetic for many years. This usage has mostly been phased out due to the risk of liver damage (often delayed) and cardiac sensitivity. Because of its toxicity and severe effects on the liver, kidneys, and central nervous system, this compound's usage as an anaesthetic has been phased out in favour of safer alternatives.

2. Most of the chloroform produced is used to make monochlorodifluoromethane ($CFCl_2H$), a refrigerant as well as an intermediary in the creation of tetrafluoroethene, which may subsequently be polymerized (PTFE). Chloroform is used to make colours, medicines, and insecticides, among other things.

3. Iodine, alkaloids, lipids, and other compounds are dissolved in trichloromethane.

4. Because of its solvent properties, chloroform is also utilised in the extraction of antibiotics, vitamins, and flavours.

   It was employed in toothpaste, mouthwash, and toothache-relieving remedies because it was 40 times sweeter than sugar and had pain-relieving effects.

5. Chloroform is used in molecular biology for a variety of purposes, including DNA extraction from cells using an extraction buffer.

6. It is utilised as a fumigant for stored-grain crops and as an intermediary in the synthesis of colours and insecticides such as chloropicrin.

7. To extract medicines from plants, chloroform is utilised.

Iodoform

Molecular formula: CHI_3

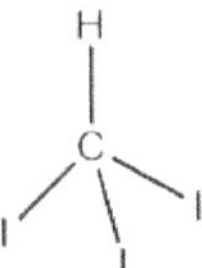

Uses:

1. Iodoform us used to treat minor skin conditions due to its antiseptic properties.

2. Due to its antimicrobial properties following topical administration, minimal levels of iodoform may be found in disinfectants and it is more primarily used for veterinary purposes.

3. Iodoform has also been found in dental paste and root canal filling materials in combination with other intracanal medications due to its radiopacity.

4. It is used as a topical anti-infective, applied to the skin.

5. It can be used in the process of removing heavy metals such as mercury from fuids.

Ethyl Chloride:

Molecular formula: CH_3CH_2Cl

Uses:

1. Medication is used to prevent pain caused by injections and minor surgical procedures. It is also used for the temporary relief of minor sports injuries. Ethyl chloride also helps to relieve deep muscle pain when used with muscle stretching techniques.
2. Chloroethane is used as recreational inhalant drug.
3. It is also used as mild anesthetic propellant as it acts as central nervous depressant.
4. It is used in dentistry it is used as a means of diagnosing a dead tooth.
5. It is used to produce tetraethyllead (TEL), an anti-knock additive for gasoline.
6. It plays an important role to treat cellulose to make ethyl cellulose, a thickening agent and binder in paints, cosmetics and similar products.

Dichloromethane:

Molecular formula: CCl_2H_2

Uses:

1. In laboratories, methylene chloride is used to extract chemicals from plants or foods for medicine such as steroids, antibiotics and vitamins.
2. Dichloromethane cleansers can clean medical equipment rapidly and effectively without creating corrosion or harm to heat-sensitive parts.
3. Dichloromethane has been recently known to exhibit anti-pyretic properties.
4. Dichloromethane is a solvent that may be used to make medicinal goods.
5. Paint stripping, pharmaceutical manufacturing, paint remover manufacturing, metal cleaning and degreasing, adhesives manufacturing and use, polyurethane foam production, film base manufacturing, polycarbonate resin production, and solvent distribution and formulation are just a few of the industries that use methylene chloride.
6. Aerosol grade methylene chloride is a more stable substance that may be used in aerosol cans, adhesives, and paint compositions. Methylene chloride is a powerful solvent, flammability suppressor, vapour pressure depressant, and viscosity thinner that is utilised in aerosols. Methylene chloride is a common solvent used in adhesive formulations because of its high dissolving power, low flammability, and quick drying time.

Tetrachloromethane

Molecular formula: CCl_4

Uses:

1. Tetrachloromethane is an effective solvent within the chemical industry and is used to clean machinery and electrical equipment.
2. Uses of tetrachloromethane/carbontetrachloride (CCl_4) as employed in the production of aerosol can refrigerants and propellants.
3. It's utilised to make chlorofluorocarbons and other compounds as a feedstock.
4. It's employed in the production of pharmaceuticals as a solvent.
5. Carbon tetrachloride was widely used as a cleaning fluid, a degreasing agent in businesses, a home spot reamer, and a fire extinguisher until the mid 1960s.
6. Tetrachloromethane/carbontetrachloride has a negative impact on the environment (CCl_4). It is concerned about the potential for harm to one's health.
7. It is extremely harmful to living things.
8. The first impact of acute CCl_4 exposure via any route is depression of the central nervous system (CNS).
    (i)   Prolonged exposure causes harm to the liver and kidneys.
    (ii) CCl_4 is a carcinogen as well. It raises your chances of getting liver cancer.

Alcohols

Alcohols are hydroxy derivatives of hydrocarbons that form a family of chemicals known as alcohols. Depending on the amount of hydroxy groups in them, they are classed as mono-, di-, or trihydric alcohols.

CH_3OH	CH_2OH | CH_2OH	CH_2OH | $CHOH$ | CH_2OH
Methyl alcohol	Glycol	Glycerol

Classification of alcohols

Monohydric alcohols (alcohols with one hydroxy group) are divided into three categories based on whether the hydroxy group is connected to a primary, secondary, or tertiary carbon atom.

(i) Primary alcohol: Primary alcohols are those in which the hydroxy group is connected to a primary carbon atom. For example:

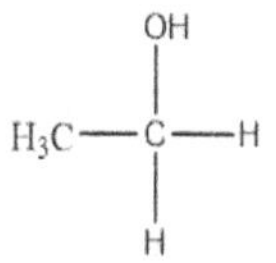

| | Ethyl alcohol | n-Propyl alcohol | Benzyl alcohol |

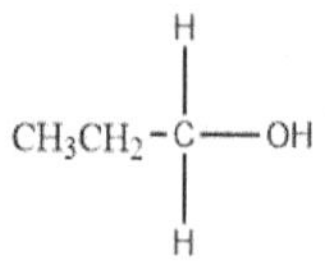

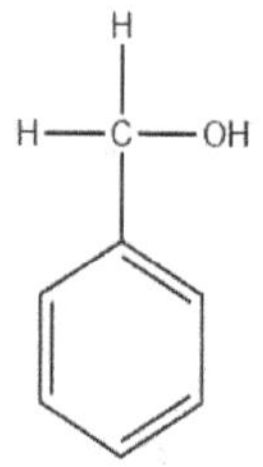

(ii) Secondary alcohol: Secondary alcohols are alcohols with a hydroxy group connected to a secondary carbon atom. For example:

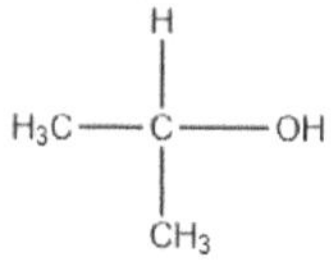

| | Isopropyl alcohol | sec.-Butyl alcohol |

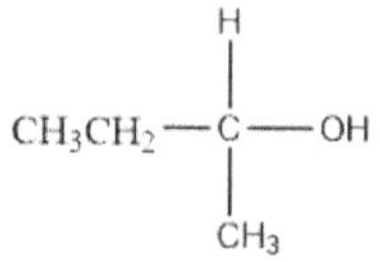

(iii) Tertiary alcohols: Tertiary alcohols are alcohols with a hydroxy group connected to a tertiary carbon atom. For example:

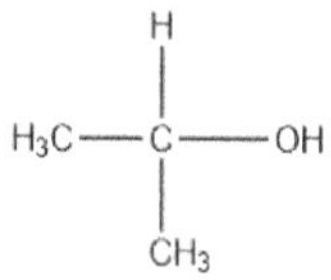

| | Isopropyl alcohol | sec.-Butyl alcohol |

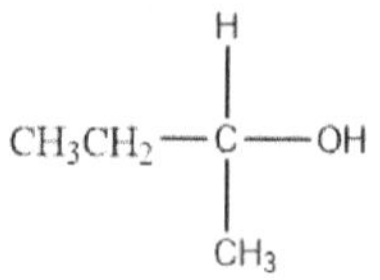

Physical Properties of Alcohols

The electrons of the C-O and O-H bons are pushed towards the oxygen atom because oxygen is more electronegative than carbon or hydrogen. Alcohols are polar substances because they include the -O-H group in their molecules. As a result, the oxygen atom has a partial negative charge, whereas the carbon and hydrogen atoms connected to it have partial positive charges.

Also, water has bent type geometry like water molecule.

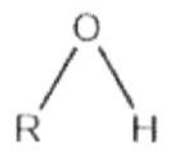

Bent geomtery

1. **Physical state**: Lower alcohols are colourless liquids with an alcoholic odour, whereas higher alcohols are waxy solids that are colourless and tasteless.

2. **Hydrogen bonding**: Intermolecular hydrogen bonding is feasible in alcohols because hydrogen atoms are bonded to electronegative oxygen atoms. Alcohols exist as linked molecules rather than simple monomeric units due to intermolecular hydrogen bonding.

3. **Boiling point**: Alcohols have a substantially higher boiling point than hydrocarbons of equal weight due to the presence of intermolecular hydrogen bonding among alcohol molecules. The substantial intermolecular hydrogen bonding inherent in alcohols necessitates a large amount of energy.

   For example,

CH_3CH_2OH	$CH_3\text{-}O\text{-}CH_3$	$CH_3CH_2CH_3$
Ethyl alcohol	Dimethyl ether	Propane
Boiling Point (K) 351.5	249	231

4. **Solubility:** Because hydrogen bonds develop between alcohol and water molecules, the lower members of alcohol are soluble in water.

   Solubility of alcohols declines as the non-polar hydrocarbon character of the molecules becomes more prevalent in comparison to the polar O-H group as the length of the hydrocarbon chain rises. As a result, the degree of hydrogen bond formation with water reduces, and hence the solubility in water decreases.

Test to Distinguish various Types of Alcohols

1. **Lucas test** is used commonly to distinguish between different types of alcohols. In Lucas test, alcohols are treated with Lucas reagent which is an equimolar mixture of conc. HCl and anhydrous Zinc Chloride. Appearance of cloudiness in the reaction mixture indicated the conversion of alcohol into alkyl chloride. Following observations have been noted:

   (i)   A tertiary alcohol reacts immediately and cloudiness appears immediately.

   (ii) Because a secondary alcohol reacts in five minutes, cloudiness arises after that time.

   (iii) Because a primary alcohol does not react much at room temperature, there is no cloudiness.

Differences between primary, secondary and tertiary alcohol:

Primary alcohol	Secondary alcohol	Tertiary alcohol
RCH_2OH $\downarrow$ $HCl/ZnCl_2$ $RCH_2Cl + H_2O$ No cloudiness at Room temperature	R_2CHOH $\downarrow$ $HCl/ZnCl_2$ $R_2CHCl + H_2O$ Cloudiness within five minutes	$R_3C\text{-}OH$ $\downarrow$ $HCl/ZnCl_2$ $R_3C\text{-}Cl + H_2O$ Cloudiness appears immediately

2. **Victor Meyer's approach** has previously been used to discriminate between different kinds of alcohols. Alcohols are treated with HI, $AgNO_2$, and NaOH in this procedure, resulting in red, blue, or colourless solutions depending on the kind of alcohol.

The procedure of Victor Meyer is as follows:

(i)   Using concentrated HI or red phosphorous and iodine, the provided alcohol is transformed into an iodide.

(ii)   To make nitroalkane, the iodide is reacted with silver nitrite.

(iii) Nitroalkane is alkaline with KOH after being treated with nitrous acid (NaNO2+H2SO4).

The original alcohol is primary if a blood red colour is achieved.

The alcohol is secondary if a blue colour is obtained.

The alcohol is tertiary if no colour is created.

Differences between primary, secondary and tertiary alcohol.

Primary alcohol	Secondary alcohol	Tertiary alcohol
RCH_2OH $\downarrow$ $P + I_2$ RCH_2I $\downarrow$ $AgNO_2$ RCH_2NO_2 $\downarrow$ $O{=}NOH$ (nitrous acid) $CH_3C{=}NOH(NO_2)$ (Nitrolic acid) Gives blood red colour with alkali	R_2CHOH $\downarrow$ $P + I_2$ R_2CHI $\downarrow$ $AgNO_2$ R_2CHNO_2 $\downarrow$ $O{=}NOH$ (nitrous acid) $R_2C(NO)(NO_2)$ (Pseudo nitrol) Gives blue colour with alkali	R_3COH $\downarrow$ $P + I_2$ R_3CI $\downarrow$ $AgNO_2$ R_3CNO_2 $\downarrow$ HONO (nitrous acid) No action No specific colour obtained

Methods of Preparation of Alcohols

1. **Reduction of carbonyl compounds:** Aldehydes and ketones can be converted to primary alcohols and secondary alcohols in a variety of methods, as shown below:

(a) Catalytic hydrogenation: By hydrogenation in the presence of a catalyst such as nickel, palladium, or platinum, aldehydes and ketones can be efficiently reduced to primary alcohols or secondary alcohols.

$$\underset{\text{Aldehyde}}{\underset{H}{\overset{R}{>}}C=O} \quad + \quad H_2 \quad \xrightarrow{\text{Ni}} \quad \underset{\text{Primary alcohol}}{RCH_2OH}$$

$$\underset{\text{Ketones}}{\underset{R'}{\overset{R}{>}}C=O} \quad + \quad H_2 \quad \xrightarrow{\text{Ni}} \quad \underset{\text{Sec. alcohol}}{\underset{R'}{\overset{R}{>}}CHOH}$$

(b) Reduction with complex metal hydrides: Complex metal hydrides such as lithium aluminium hydride (LiAlH$_0$) and sodium borohydride can also be used to convert aldehydes and ketones to alcohols (NaBH$_4$).

$$\underset{\text{Propanal}}{CH_3CH_2CHO} \quad \xrightarrow[\text{(ii) } H_3O^+]{\text{(i) NaBH}_4, \text{ ethanol}} \quad \underset{\text{Propan-1-ol}}{CH_3CH_2CH_2OH}$$

$$\underset{\text{Butan-2-one}}{CH_3CH_2-\overset{\overset{\displaystyle O}{\|}}{C}CH_3} \quad \xrightarrow[\text{(ii) } H_3O^+]{\text{(i) LiAlH}_4, \text{ ether}} \quad \underset{\text{Butan-2-ol}}{CH_3CH_2CHOHCH_3}$$

It has been observed that one mole of LiAlH$_4$ or NaBH$_4$ reduces four moles of aldehyde or ketone.

2. **Reduction of carboxylic acids and esters**: Lithium aluminium hydride can be used to reduce carboxylic acids and esters to produce primary alcohols (LiAlH4).

$$\underset{\text{Carboxylic acid}}{R-\overset{\overset{\displaystyle O}{\|}}{C}-OH} \quad \xrightarrow[\text{(ii) } H_3O^+]{\text{(i) LiAlH}_4} \quad \underset{\text{Primary alcohol}}{R-CH_2OH}$$

$$\underset{\text{Butan-1-oic acid}}{CH_3CH_2CH_2COOH} \quad \xrightarrow[\text{(ii) } H_3O^+]{\text{(i) LiAlH}_4} \quad \underset{\text{1-Butanol}}{CH_3CH_2CH_2CH_2OH}$$

$$R-\overset{\overset{\displaystyle O}{\parallel}}{C}-OR' \xrightarrow[\text{(ii) } H_3O^+]{\text{(i) LiAlH}_4} RCH_2OH \quad + \quad R'OH$$

$$CH_3CH_2CH_2\overset{\overset{\displaystyle O}{\parallel}}{C}-OC_2H_5 \xrightarrow[\text{(ii) } H_3O^+]{\text{(i) LiAlH}_4} CH_3CH_2CH_2CH_2OH \quad + \quad C_2H_5OH$$

Ethyl butyrate   1-Butanol   Ethanol

3. **Direct hydration of alkenes**: In the presence of acids such as sulphuric acid and phosphoric acid, water is added across reactive alkenes to form alcohols, according to Markownikoff's rule.

Alkene   + $H_2O \xrightarrow{H^+}$ Alcohol

$$CH_3-\overset{\overset{\displaystyle CH_3}{|}}{C}=CH_2 \quad + \quad H_2O \xrightarrow{H^+} H_3C-\overset{\overset{\displaystyle CH_3}{|}}{\underset{\underset{\displaystyle CH_3}{|}}{C}}-OH$$

2-Methyl propene   tert-Butyl alcohol

4. **Oxymercuration-demercuration of alkenes**: Alkenes for organo mercurial compounds are treated with mercuric acetate in a water-tetrahydrofuran solution in this procedure. Sodium borohydride (NaBH4) is used to further decrease these compounds, yielding alcohols.

$$\text{Alkene} + H_2O + Hg(OOCH_3)_2 \xrightarrow[\text{(Oxymercuration)}]{\text{THF}} \text{Organomercurial Compound} + CH_3COOH$$

Alkene   Mercuric acetate

$$\xrightarrow[\text{(Demercuration)}]{\text{NaBH}_4} \text{Alcohol} \quad + \quad Hg \quad + \quad CH_3COO^-$$

Alcohol

Water and mercuric acetate are added to the double bond in the first stage. Oxymercuration is the name for this process. The mercuric acetate group is replaced by hydrogen in the second step, which involves treating the organomercurial molecule with sodium borohydride. Demercuration is the term for this.

5. **Hydroboration-oxidation of alkenes**: Alkenes are hydroborated to generate alkyl boranes when they are treated with diborane (BH3)2. In an alkaline solution, hydrogen peroxide quickly oxidises the alkyl boranes to produce alcohols.

$$H_2C\!\!=\!\!CH_2 \;+\; (BH_3)_2 \longrightarrow CH_3CH_2BH_2 \xrightarrow{CH_2=CH_2} (CH_3CH_2)_2BH$$

Ethylene   ethylborane   Diethylborane

$$\downarrow CH_2=CH_2$$

$$3CH_3CH_2OH \;+\; H_3BO_3 \xleftarrow{OH^-} 3H_2O_2 + (CH_3CH_2)_3B$$

ethyl alcohol   triethylborane

Hydroboration-oxidation is also a regioselective reaction and the alcohol obtained is such as if anti-Markownikoff addition of water to alkenes had taken place. Thus this method can be used for the preparation of alcohols which cannot be prepared by other methods of hydration of alkenes.

6. **Grignard synthesis**: This is the most important method for the preparation of primary, secondary and tertiary alcohols which involves the reaction of carbonyl compound (aldehyde or ketone) with Grignard's reagent (RMgX). The addition product obtained initially is decomposed with water in the presence of acids such as HCl or H_2SO_4, to get alcohols.

$$\begin{array}{c}\diagdown\\C=O\\\diagup\end{array} \;+\; RMgX \xrightarrow{\text{Dry ether}} -\!\!\overset{|}{\underset{\underset{R}{|}}{C}}\!\!-OMgX$$

Carbonyl compound   Griganrd reagent   Addition product

$$\downarrow \begin{array}{l}H_3O^+\\ -Mg(OH)X\end{array}$$

$$-\!\!\overset{|}{\underset{\underset{R}{|}}{C}}\!\!-OH$$

Alcohol

(i) The ultimate result of the aforementioned reaction is a secondary alcohol if the carbonyl molecule utilised is an aldehyde (other than formaldehyde).

Aldehyde → Secondary alcohol

$$R'\text{—CHO} \xrightarrow[\text{(Dry ether)}]{RMgX} R'\text{—CH(OMgX)}\text{—R} \longrightarrow R'\text{—CH(OH)}\text{—R}$$

Acetaldehyde → Isopropyl alcohol

$$CH_3\text{—CHO} \xrightarrow[\text{(Dry ether)}]{CH_3MgX} CH_3\text{—CH(OMgI)}\text{—CH}_3 \longrightarrow CH_3\text{—CH(OH)}\text{—CH}_3$$

(ii) The production of tertiary alcohol occurs when ketone is treated with Grignard reagent.

Ketone → Tertiary alcohol

$$R'\text{—C(R'')=O} \xrightarrow[\text{(Dry ether)}]{RMgX} R'\text{—C(R'')(OMgX)}\text{—R} \longrightarrow R'\text{—C(R'')(OH)}\text{—R}$$

Acetone → tert-Butyl alcohol

$$CH_3\text{—C(CH}_3\text{)=O} \xrightarrow[\text{(Dry ether)}]{CH_3MgX} CH_3\text{—C(CH}_3\text{)(OMgI)}\text{—CH}_3 \longrightarrow CH_3\text{—C(CH}_3\text{)(OH)}\text{—CH}_3$$

8. By the hydrolysis of alkyl halides: Alkyl halides form corresponding alcohols on boiling with aqueous alkali solution or with most silver oxide.

$$\underset{\text{Alkyl halide}}{R\text{-X}} + K^-OH^-(aq) \xrightarrow{\text{boil}} \underset{\text{Alcohol}}{R\text{-OH}} + KX$$

$$\underset{\text{Bromoethane}}{C_2H_5\text{-Br}} + K^-OH^-(aq) \xrightarrow{\text{boil}} \underset{\text{Ethanol}}{C_2H_5\text{-OH}} + KBr$$

$$\underset{\substack{\text{Iodomethane moist silver} \\ \text{oxide}}}{C_2H_5\text{-I} + Ag^+OH^-} \xrightarrow{\text{boil}} \underset{\text{Ethanol}}{C_2H_5OH} + AgI$$

7. **By hydrolysis of esters:** The hydrolysis of esters with an alkali solution is a typical method for making alcohols from natural esters.

$$RCOOR' + NaOH \longrightarrow RCOONa + R'OH$$

Ester   aq   Sodium salt of acid   Alcohol

$$C_{15}H_{31}COOC_{16}H_{33} + NaOH \longrightarrow C_{15}H_{31}COONa + C_{16}H_{33}OH$$

Cetyl palmitate   aq   Sodium palmitate   Cetyl alcohol

Alcohols undergo variety of reactions due to hydroxyl group present in them which are as follows:

Chemical Properties of Alcohols

(i)   Reactions involving the cleavage of O-H bond, i.e., RO-H.

(ii)   Cleavage-of-the-C-OH-bond reactions, i.e., R-OH.

(iii)   Reactions involving both alkyl and hydroxyl groups of the alcohol molecules.

Reactions involving the cleavage of O-H bond.

In these types of reactions, the usual sequence of reactivity of alcohols is:

Primary alcohol > Secondary alcohol > Tertiary alcohol.

The aforementioned sequence may be interpreted as O pulling the shared pair of electrons towards itself during the cleavage of the O-H bond, resulting in negative charge. The electron releasing (+I) inductive action of the alkyl group may now be used to explain the relative order of reactivity. The number of alkyl groups connected to the carbon transporting the O-H group grows from one to three as we progress from primary to secondary to tertiary alcohols. The negative charge on the O atom increases as the number of alkyl groups increases due to the electron releasing action of alkyl groups.

As a result, the electrons in the O-H bond cannot be pulled far enough towards oxygen, and the ease with which the O-H bond may be cleaved reduces. Thus, the order of reactivity in reactions involving the cleavage of O-H bond is:

Primary alcohol > Secondary alcohol > Tertiary alcohol.

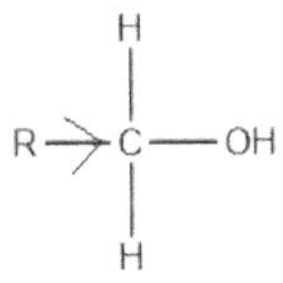

Primary alcohol 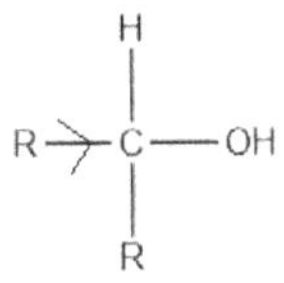   Secondary Alcohol 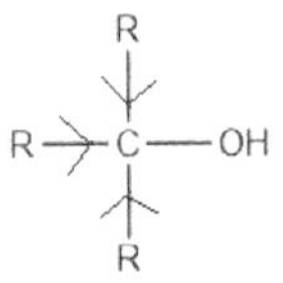   Tertairy Alcohol

1. **Reaction with metals:** Alcohols release hydrogen and generate metal alkoxides when they react with active metals including sodium, potassium, magnesium, and aluminium.

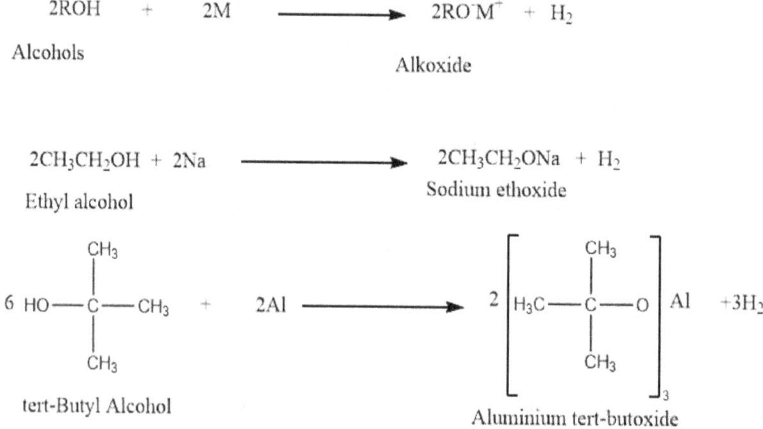

$$2ROH \; + \; 2M \longrightarrow 2RO^-M^+ \; + \; H_2$$

Alcohols → Alkoxide

$$2CH_3CH_2OH + 2Na \longrightarrow 2CH_3CH_2ONa + H_2$$

Ethyl alcohol → Sodium ethoxide

tert-Butyl Alcohol → Aluminium tert-butoxide

From the above reactions it is quite clear that alcohols are acidic in nature as the -OH group contains highly electronegative oxygen attached to hydrogen. The O-H bond is polarized in character and allows the separation of hydrogen as H^+ ion.

2. **Reaction with Grignard reagent:** Alcohols produce hydrocarbons when they react with Grignard reagent.

$$R'OH \; + \; RMgX \longrightarrow RH \; + \; R'OMgX$$

Alcohol   Grignard reagent   Hydrocarbon

$$CH_3OH \; + \; C_2H_5MgI \longrightarrow C_2H_6 \; + \; CH_3OMgI$$

Methyl alcohol   Ethyl magnesium iodide   Ethane

3. **Reaction with organic acids:** Esters are formed when alcohols combine with organic acids. Esterification is a process that takes place in the presence of strong sulphuric acid or hydrogen chloride gas.

$$R-\overset{O}{\overset{\|}{C}}-OH + HOR' \underset{}{\overset{conc.H_2SO_4}{\rightleftharpoons}} RCOOR' + H_2O$$

Acid   Alcohol   Ester

$$CH_3-\overset{O}{\overset{\|}{C}}-OH + HOC_2H_5 \rightleftharpoons CH_3COOC_2H_5 + H_2O$$

Acetic acid   Ethyl alcohol   Ethyl acetate

Mechanism: The first protonation of the carbonyl oxygen of the carboxylic acid by the proton produced by the acid is the mechanism of esterification. As a result, the carbonyl carbon becomes positively charged and is easily nucleophilized by the alcohols' oxygen.

Relative reactivities of alcohols and acids: The steric barrier produced by the presence of big groups in alcohols and carboxylic acids has a significant impact on their respective reactivities in esterification. The rate of esterification is slowed when the size of groups around the -OH group of the alcohol or the -COOH group of the acid increases. As a result, the following is the decreasing rate of esterification of various alcohols and acids:

Alcohols: $CH_3OH > CH_3CH_2OH > (CH_3)_2CHOH > (CH_3)_3COH$

Carboxylic acids: $HCOOH > CH_3COOH > (CH_3)_2CHCOOH > (CH_3)_3CCOOH$

4. **Reaction with acid halides or acid anhydrides**: When alcohols are treated with acid halides or acid anhydrides, the hydrogen atom is replaced by an acyl group (RCO-), and an ester is generated as a result. Acylation is the name for this process.

$$CH_3COCl + HOC_2H_5 \longrightarrow CH_3COOC_2H_5 + HCl$$

Acetyl chloride   Ethanol   Ethyl acetate

$$CH_3COOC_2H_5 + CH_3COOH$$

Acetic anhydride   Ethanol   Ethyl acetate   Acetic acid

Reactions involving the cleavage of C-OH bond

The following is the sequence of reactions involving the cleavage of the C-OH bond:

Tertiary alcohol > Secondary alcohol > Primary alcohol

The +I effect of alkyl groups explains the aforementioned order. As we progress from primary to tertiary alcohols, the number of alkyl groups increases from one to three. As the number of alkyl groups linked to the carbon bearing the -OH group grows, more electrons are pushed towards oxygen, causing the C-OH bond to become more polar and reactive. As a result, tertiary alcohols, secondary alcohols, and primary alcohols are the most reactive.

5. **Reaction with hydrogen halides**: Alkyl halides and water are formed when alcohols combine with hydrogen halides.

$$ROH + HX \longrightarrow RX + H_2O$$
Alcohol   Alkyl halide

$$C_2H_5OH + HCl\,(g) \xrightarrow{\text{anhydrous } ZnCl_2} C_2H_5Cl + H_2O$$
Ethyl alcohol   Ethyl chloride

The order of reactivity of halogen acids is HI > HBr > HCl

6. **Reaction with phosphorus halides**: Alcohols produce alkyl halides when they react with phosphorus halides such as PCl_5, PCl_3, PBr_3, or PI_3.

$$ROH + PCl_5 \longrightarrow RCl + POCl_3 + HCl$$
Alcohol   Alkyl chloride

$$3ROH + PX_3 \longrightarrow 3RX + H_3PO_3$$
Alcohol   Alkyl halide

Benzyl alcohol + $PCl_5 \longrightarrow$ Benzyl chloride + $POCl_3$ + HCl

$$3C_2H_5OH + PI_3 \longrightarrow 3C_2H_5I + H_3PO_3$$
Ethyl chloride   Ethyl iodide

7. **Reaction with thionyl chloride**: Alkyl chlorides are formed when alcohols react with thionyl chloride in the presence of a base, such as a tertiary amine. Alcohols can also be made into alkyl chloride by refluxing them with thionyl chloride in the presence of pyridine. Darzen's response is another name for this response.

$$CH_3CH_2OH + SOCl_2 \xrightarrow{\text{pyridine}} CH_3CH_2Cl + SO_2 + HCl$$
chloroethane

Reactions involving both alkyl and hydroxyl groups

1. **Acidic dehydration:** When alcohols are heated with sulphuric acid, phosphoric acid or boric acid, alcohols get dehydrated to form alkenes.

$$CH_3CH_2OH \xrightarrow{H_2SO_4(433K)} CH_2{=}CH_2 + H_2O$$

Ethyl alcohol → Ethylene

$$CH_3CH_2CH_2CH_2OH \xrightarrow[-H_2O]{H_2SO_4} CH_3CH{=}CHCH_3 \;+\; CH_3CH_2CH{=}CH_2$$

n-Butyl alcohol → 2-Butene (Main product) + 1-Butene (Minor product)

Mechanism of dehydration: The dehydration of alcohols is believed to take place in three steps.

The three steps involved in dehydration of alcohols is as follows:

1. In the first step, alcohol combines with a proton (H^+) released by acid to form protonated alcohols or oxonium ion.

2. Protonated alcohol loses a molecule of water in the next step to generate carbocation.

3. In the last step, the carbocation loses a proton molecule to form alkene.

The various steps discussed above are summarized as follows:

(1) Ethyl alcohol $+$ H^+ ⇌ Protonated alcohol or oxonium ion

(2) ⇌ (Rate determining step) Carbocation $+$ H_2O

(3) ⇌ $H_2C{=}CH_2$ $+$ H^+ (Ethylene)

Relative ease of dehydration of alcohols: The relative ease of dehydration of different kinds of alcohols has been reported to follow the following order:

Tertiary alcohol > Secondary alcohol > Primary alcohol

On the basis of the creation of carbocation in step 1, the aforementioned sequence of reactivity may be explained (2). Phase (2), which involves the production of carbocation, is the rate-determining step in the overall reaction. Furthermore, the relative stability order of different carbocations is as follows:

Tertiary carbocation> Secondary carbocation> Primary carbocation

Hence, reaction resulting in the formation of tertiary carbocation will be fastest followed by the reaction resulting in the formation of secondary carbocation and slowest in those reactions resulting in the formation of primary carbocations.

As a result, the above order of ease of dehydration of alcohols is the same as the order of ease of production of carbocations:

Tertiary alcohol > Secondary alcohol > Primary alcohol

Orientation of dehydration: Dehydration of various alcohols produces a variety of isomeric alkenes. The ratio of alkenes produced in a reaction is determined by the reaction circumstances. In line with Saytzeff's rule, dehydration of an alcohol promotes the creation of more stable alkenes.

$$CH_3\text{-}CH_2\text{-}CHOH\text{-}CH_3 \xrightarrow[-H_2O]{H_3PO_3\text{-}Al_2O_3,\ 298K}$$

$CH_3\text{-}CH_2\text{-}CH{=}CH_2$
1-Butene (24.1%)
(less stable)

$+$

$CH_3\text{-}CH{=}CHCH_3$
2-Butene(75.9%)
(more stable)

The major product is more stable than the other since it is more highly substituted.

Rearrangement of carbocations and formation of unexpected products during dehydration:

It has been experimentally found that during dehydration of alcohols alkenes formed as product are not what one would normally expect as the position of double bond or sometimes even the carbon skeleton may be quite unexpected.

For example, consider dehydration of n-butyl alcohol gives a mixture of 2-butene (main product) and 1-butene whereas normally only 1-butene is expected.

$$CH_3\text{-}CH_2\text{-}CH_2\text{-}CH_2OH \xrightarrow[-H_2O]{H_3PO_3\text{-}Al_2O_3,\ 298K}$$

$CH_3\text{-}CH_2\text{-}CH{=}CH_2$
1-Butene

$+$

$CH_3\text{-}CH{=}CHCH_3$

2-Butene
(Unexpected but major product)

The formation of 2-butene can be described in terms of intermediate carbocation rearrangement. Primary carbocations rearrange to generate secondary carbocations, and secondary carbocations rearrange to generate tertiary carbocations, according to research. The migration of a hydride ion (hydrogen atom plus two bonding electrons) from a neighbouring carbon atom to the positively charged carbon of the carbocation is typical of rearrangement in the aforementioned situation. Hydride shift is the term for this type of migration.

Rearrangement can also occur when an alkyl group with its pair of bonding electrons migrates from a positively charged carbon next to it. Alkyl shift is the term for this sort of migration. These migrations are also known as 1,2-shifts since they occur on nearby carbon atoms.

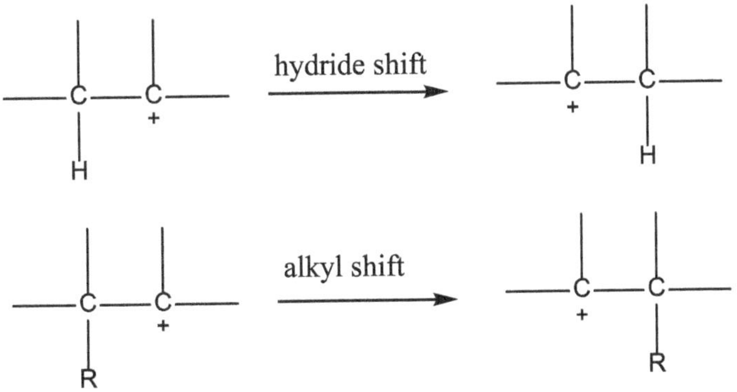

Example of hydride shift: The intermediate primary carbocation created during dehydration of n-Butyl alcohol is n-butyl carbocation, which undergoes a 1,2-hydride shift to generate the more stable sec-butyl ion. After rearrangement, the carbocation loses an H+ ion, forming the more stable 2-butene as the preferred product.

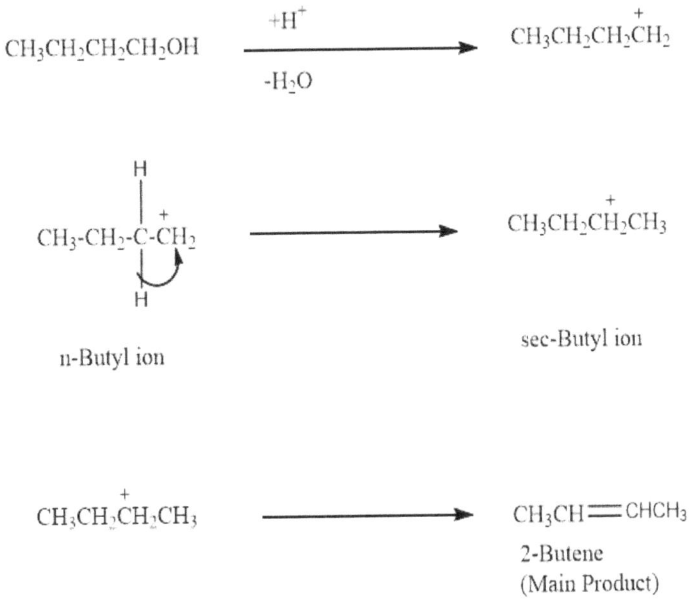

$$CH_3CH_2CH_2CH_2OH \xrightarrow[-H_2O]{+H^+} CH_3CH_2CH_2\overset{+}{C}H_2$$

n-Butyl ion

sec-Butyl ion

$$CH_3CH_2\overset{+}{C}H_2CH_3 \longrightarrow CH_3CH=CHCH_3$$

2-Butene
(Main Product)

2. **Oxidation**: Alcohol oxidation can be accomplished with a number of reagents, including acidified or alkaline potassium permanganate, acidified sodium or potassium dichromate, dilute nitric acid, or CrO3 in pyridine.

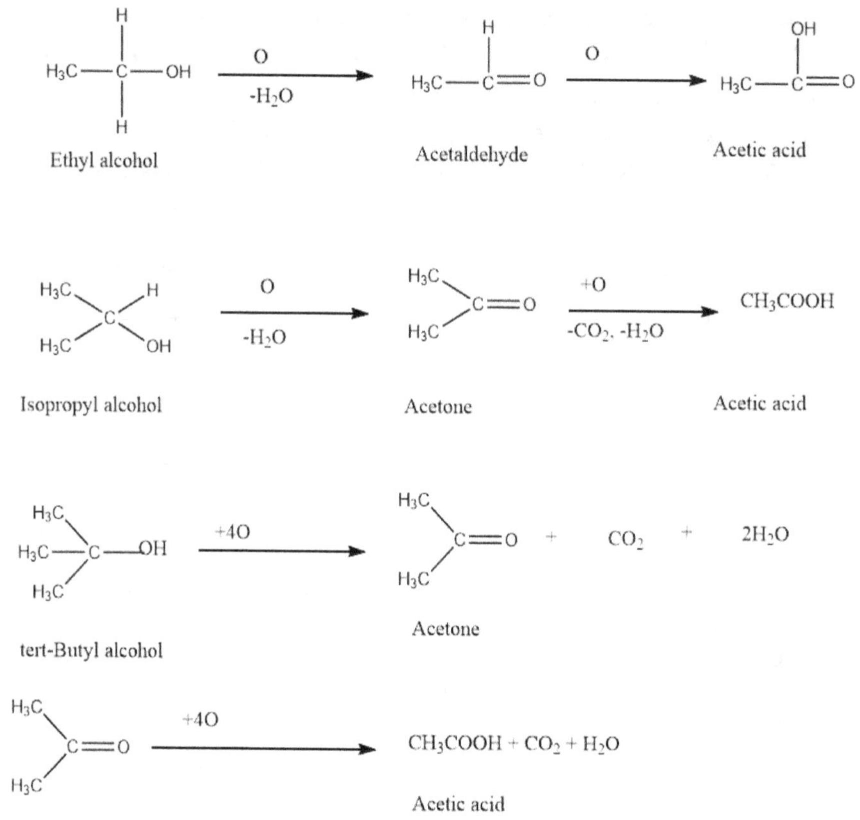

$$\underset{\text{Ethyl alcohol}}{H_3C-\overset{\overset{\displaystyle H}{|}}{\underset{\underset{\displaystyle H}{|}}{C}}-OH} \xrightarrow[-H_2O]{O} \underset{\text{Acetaldehyde}}{H_3C-\overset{\overset{\displaystyle H}{|}}{C}=O} \xrightarrow{O} \underset{\text{Acetic acid}}{H_3C-\overset{\overset{\displaystyle OH}{|}}{C}=O}$$

$$\underset{\text{Isopropyl alcohol}}{\overset{\displaystyle H_3C}{\underset{\displaystyle H_3C}{}}\!\!>\!\!\overset{\displaystyle H}{\underset{\displaystyle OH}{C}}} \xrightarrow{-H_2O} \underset{\text{Acetone}}{\overset{\displaystyle H_3C}{\underset{\displaystyle H_3C}{}}\!\!>\!\!C=O} \xrightarrow[-CO_2,\,-H_2O]{+O} \underset{\text{Acetic acid}}{CH_3COOH}$$

$$\underset{\text{tert-Butyl alcohol}}{\overset{\displaystyle H_3C}{\underset{\displaystyle H_3C}{}}\!\!>\!\!\underset{\displaystyle H_3C}{C}-OH} \xrightarrow{+4O} \underset{\text{Acetone}}{\overset{\displaystyle H_3C}{\underset{\displaystyle H_3C}{}}\!\!>\!\!C=O} \;+\; CO_2 \;+\; 2H_2O$$

$$\overset{\displaystyle H_3C}{\underset{\displaystyle H_3C}{}}\!\!>\!\!C=O \xrightarrow{+4O} \underset{\text{Acetic acid}}{CH_3COOH + CO_2 + H_2O}$$

Different products are obtained depending on type of alcohol used.

Primary alcohols are oxidised to aldehydes, which are subsequently oxidised to acid with the same number of carbon atoms as the original alcohol.

Secondary alcohols are oxidised to yield ketones with the same number of carbon atoms as primary alcohols. Ketones are further oxidised under extreme circumstances to produce acids with fewer carbon atoms.

Tertiary alcohols, on the other hand, do not oxidise in neutral or alkaline solutions.

Tertiary alcohols are oxidised to ketones and acids with fewer carbon atoms than the reactant alcohol in the presence of acidic oxidising agents.

3. **Action of hot reduced copper**: When alcohol vapours are passed over reduced copper at high temperatures, they produce a variety of compounds.

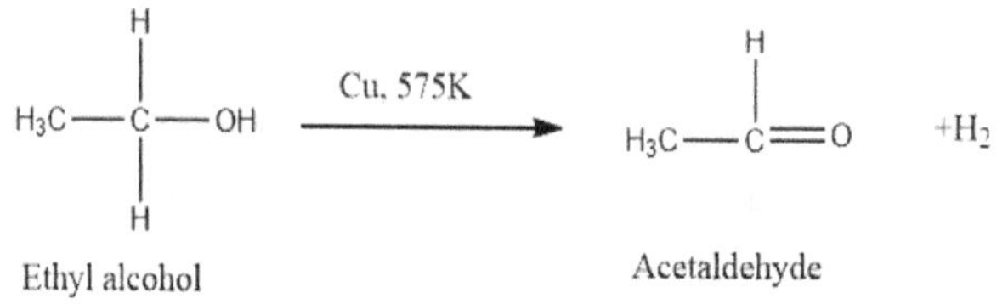

$$\underset{\text{Ethyl alcohol}}{H_3C-\overset{\overset{\displaystyle H}{|}}{\underset{\underset{\displaystyle H}{|}}{C}}-OH} \xrightarrow{Cu,\ 575K} \underset{\text{Acetaldehyde}}{H_3C-\overset{\overset{\displaystyle H}{|}}{C}=O} \quad +H_2$$

$$H_3C \diagdown \!\!\!\!\!\underset{\underset{H_3C}{|}}{\overset{H}{\underset{|}{C}}}\!\!\!\!\!\diagup OH \quad \xrightarrow{\text{Cu, 575K}} \quad H_3C \diagdown \!\!\!\!\! \underset{H_3C}{\overset{}{C}} \!\!\!\!\! = O \quad + \quad H_2$$

Isopropyl alcohol   Acetone

$$H_3C \diagdown \!\!\!\! \underset{\underset{H_3C}{|}}{\overset{}{C}} \!\!\!\! - OH \quad \xrightarrow{\text{Cu, 575K}} \quad H_3C - \overset{\overset{CH_3}{|}}{C} = CH_2 \quad + \quad H_2O$$

tert-Butyl alcohol   Iso-butylene

Qualitative Test of Alcohols

1. **Reaction with sodium metal:** Alcohols react with active metals such as sodium, potassium, magnesium and aluminium to liberate hydrogen and form metal alkoxides.

   Thus, liberation of hydrogen gas indicates the unknown same contains alcohols.

   $$2ROH \quad + \quad 2M \quad \longrightarrow \quad 2RO^-M^+ \; + \; H_2$$

   Alcohols   Alkoxide

   $$2CH_3CH_2OH + 2Na \quad \longrightarrow \quad 2CH_3CH_2ONa \; + \; H_2$$

   Ethyl alcohol   Sodium ethoxide

   $$6\; HO - \overset{\overset{CH_3}{|}}{\underset{\underset{CH_3}{|}}{C}} - CH_3 \quad + \quad 2Al \quad \longrightarrow \quad 2 \left[H_3C - \overset{\overset{CH_3}{|}}{\underset{\underset{CH_3}{|}}{C}} - O \right]_3 Al \quad +3H_2$$

   tert-Butyl Alcohol   Aluminium tert-butoxide

2. **Ester formation:** Alcohols react with organic acids to form esters. This reaction is known as esterification and is carried out in the presence of concentrated sulphuric acid or hydrogen chloride gas.

   $$R - \overset{\overset{O}{\|}}{C} - OH \; + \; HOR' \quad \underset{\longleftarrow}{\overset{\text{conc.}H_2SO_4}{\longrightarrow}} \quad RCOOR' \; + \; H_2O$$

   Acid   Alcohol   Ester

   $$CH_3 - \overset{\overset{O}{\|}}{C} - OH \; + \; HOC_2H_5 \quad \rightleftharpoons \quad CH_3COOC_2H_5 \; + \; H_2O$$

   Acetic acid   Ethyl alcohol   Ethyl acetate

Liberation of fruity smell due to ester formation indicates the unknown compound contains alcohol.

3. **Reaction with ceric ammonium nitrate**: Alcohols cause a colour shift red coloured complex when they combine with ceric ammonium nitrate reagent. This is an excellent experiment for detecting the presence of alcohol. As a result, the presence of an alcohol group is indicated by the production of (alkoxy cerium derivative) magenta colour.

$$R\text{-}OH \ + \ (NH_4)_2 \left[Ce(NO_3)_6 \right] \longrightarrow \left[ROCe(NO_3)_5 \right]^{2-}$$

Alcohol   Ceric ammonium nitrate   an alkoxy cerium(IV) derivative

Structure and Uses of Alcohols

Ethyl alcohol:CH_3CH_2OH

1. Ethanol may be found in a wide range of cosmetics and beauty products. It may be used as an astringent to help clean the skin, as a lotion preservative to keep the contents from separating, and as a hairspray adherer.

2. Ethanol is a common ingredient in many hand sanitizers because it is efficient in killing germs like bacteria, fungi, and viruses.

3. Ethanol can help to uniformly distribute food colouring and improve the flavour of food extracts. Vanilla extract is a common culinary flavouring that is made by curing and processing vanilla beans in an ethanol and water solution.

4. Ethanol is used in gasoline to help oxygenate the fuel and reduce pollution. Ethanol is usually found in a blend known as E10, which is composed of 10% ethanol and 90% gasoline.

5. Because it rapidly mixes with water and many organic compounds, ethanol is an excellent solvent for paints, lacquers, and varnishes, as well as personal care and household cleaning products. Ethanol is also used as a preservative in cleaning solutions since it is effective at destroying germs that are potentially hazardous to humans.

Methanol: CH_3OH

1. Methanol is commonly used as a component in the production of formaldehyde. This methanol-derived compound is widely utilised in the manufacture of plastics, such as those used in building materials, automobile components, paints, explosives, and wrinkle-resistant artificial textiles. Morticians and scientists use formaldehyde to preserve corpses and laboratory materials.

2. Methanol may be used to generate acetic acid, dimethyl ether, and propylene, which is used in antifreeze, among other important solvents. Methanol can also be included in anti-freeze products.

3. Methanol may be used as a fuel in both gasoline and biodiesel cars. Because of its great flammability and use as a solvent, it can aid in the mixing and ignition of other fuels.

4. Methanol is also utilised in the manufacturing of polyester textiles and fibres, acrylic plastics, insecticides, textile solvents, medicines, and windshield wiper fluid in industry.

5. It's utilised in the production of cholesterol, streptomycin, vitamins, hormones, and other medications as a solvent.

6. It's also utilised as a solvent in the pharmaceutical industry, and because it's a polar liquid at room temperature, it's employed as an antifreeze and ethanol denaturant.

Chlorobutanol

Molecular formula: $C_4H_7OCl_3$

1. Pet enthusiasts use chlorobutanol mixed with water as humane method of euthanizing reptiles.

2. Chlorobutanol, also known as trichloro-2-methyl-2-propane, is a chemical preservative often found in a variety of cosmetic and medicinal items.

3. Chlorobutanol is used to treat, control, prevent, and alleviate the symptoms of the following illnesses and conditions:
   - Mild skin soreness
   - Scratches
   - Grazes
   - Dental plaque formation
   - Gingivitis
   - Oral hygiene
   - Mouth ulceration
   - Candida infections in the mouthThroat infections
   - Cold relief

4. Chlorobutanol has been used in anesthesia and euthanasia of invertebrates and fishes.

5. Chlorobutanol may be used as a pharmaceutical reference standard for the determination of the analyte in pharmaceutical formulations and ophthalmic ointments by various chromategraphy techniques.

Cetosteryl Alcohol

$$n = 14 \text{ to } 16$$

Cetostearyl Alcohol is a blend of cetyl and stearyl alcohols derived from either natural or synthetic sources. It's considered a fatty alcohol. Cetostearyl alcohol comes in the form of flakes that are white, waxy, and solid.

1. The following illnesses, disorders, and symptoms are treated, controlled, prevented, and improved by cetosteryl alcohol:

   - Dry skin

   - Diaper rash

   - Skin burns from radiation therapy

   - Skin irritations

2. Cetostearyl alcohol is used as an emulsion stabiliser, opacifying agent, surfactant - foam booster, and viscosity enhancing agent in the pharmaceutical and cosmetics industries. It's frequently found in creams and lotions.

3. They're found in skin lotions, hair treatments, and creams, among other things. They aid in the creation of creams that are smoother, thicker lotions, and more stable foam products.

Glycerol

Molecular formula: $C_3O_2H_8$

$$
\begin{array}{l}
CH_2OH \\
\mid \\
CHOH \\
\mid \\
CH_2OH
\end{array}
$$

1. Glycerol can be used to heal wounds and certain forms of burns due to its antiviral and antibacterial characteristics. Treatment of wounds with an 86 percent glycerol solution has also been recommended as a way to minimise inflammation in the damaged region.

2. Because of its antibacterial properties, glycerol is used in the manufacture of a variety of personal care goods, including shaving cream, toothpastes, mouthwashes, soaps, skin care products, and hair care products.

3. Glycerol is a substance used to preserve red blood cells (also known as RBCs) before they are frozen for storage.

4. Glycerol is frequently utilised as a humectant in the food sector. It's also used as a solvent and a sweetening ingredient in a variety of foods and drinks. Furthermore, this molecule is known to be utilised as a filler in low-fat meals sold commercially, such as cookies.

5. In the manufacture of various liqueurs, glycerol is occasionally used as a thickening agent. For the preservation of particular plant leaves, a solution of water and glycerol can be used.

6. Its usage as an economically significant chemical dates back to its employment in the manufacture of dynamite. The discovery and exploitation of subterranean resources, as well as the development of infrastructure, required dynamite. As a result, it accelerated the growth of industry.

7. In the pharmaceutical sector, glycerol is used to increase smoothness and flavour. It's utilised in the manufacture of tablets to make them easier to swallow. Within the body, the covering may dissolve. Glycerol is commonly used in cough lozenges to give them a sweet flavour. Glycerol suppositories can work as laxatives because they irritate the anal mucosa.

Benzyl alcohol:

Molecular formula: C_7H_8O

1. It is employed in the production of various benzyl compounds, as well as in fragrance and flavouring.
2. It is a medicinal medicine that is used to treat head lice as an anti-parasite medicine.
3. In many injectable medications, benzyl alcohol is utilised as a preservative.
4. Benzyl alcohol stops lice from sealing their spiracles, causing them to suffocate and die within ten minutes.
5. A 10% benzyl alcohol solution can be utilised as a local anaesthetic as well as an antibacterial agent.
6. This substance is found in liquid mixes used in electronic cigarettes (it enhances the flavour).
7. Benzyl alcohol may be used as a dielectric solvent for dielectrophoresis to reconfigure certain nanowires.
8. Because of its antifungal and antibacterial characteristics, it is used in the production of soaps, shampoos, and skin creams.

Propylene glycol

Molecular formula: $C_3H_8O_2$

1. Propylene glycol is a moisturiser that is used to treat or prevent dry, rough, scaly, itchy, and irritated skin, as well as mild skin irritations (e.g., diaper rash, skin burns from radiation therapy). Emollients soften and hydrate the skin while also reducing irritation and peeling. Some products (for example, zinc oxide and white petrolatum) are primarily used to protect the skin from irritation (e.g., from wetness).
2. In topical, oral, and injectable pharmaceuticals, propylene glycol is a frequent drug solubilizer. It's utilised as a vitamin stabiliser and a water-miscible cosolvent.
3. Propylene glycol is also used in cosmetics as a moisturiser and as a scent dispersion.
4. Humectant, which adds moisture and flavour.
5. Solvent, stabiliser, and preservative to extend the life of the feed.

6. Additive to provide additional energy.

7. For beverages, biscuits, cakes, and sweets, a solvent and carrier for flavour and colour in food and beverage manufacturing operations.

MCQs

1. Consider the following reaction

$$C_2H_5OH \ + \ H_2SO_4 \ \longrightarrow \ \text{Product}$$

   Among the following which one cannot be formed as a product under any conditions

   (a) Ethylene

   (b) Ethyl-hydrogen sulphate

   (c) Diethyl ether

   (d) Acetylene

2. From amongst the following alcohols the one that would react fastest with conc. HCl and anhydrous $ZnCl_2$ is:-

   (a) 2-Methyl propan-2-ol

   (b) 2-Butanol

   (c) 1-Butanol

   (d) 2-Methylpropanol

3. In the following sequence of reaction:-

$$CH_3CH_2OH \xrightarrow{P+I_2} A \xrightarrow[\text{Ether}]{Mg} B \xrightarrow{HCHO} C \xrightarrow{H_2O} D$$

   The compound 'D' is

   (a) Butanol

   (b) n-butyl alcohol

   (c) n-propyl alcohol

   (d) propanal

4. In Williamson's synthesis

   (a) An alcohol heated with conc. H_2SO_4 at 140°C

   (b) An alkyl halide is treated with sodium

   (c) An alkyl halide is treated with sodium alkoxide

   (d) None of the above

5. Primary alcohol have boiling points that are ……………..the corresponding aldehydes.

   (a) Lower than

   (b) Higher than

   (c) About the same

   (d) Not easy to compare

6. Silver acetate reacts with Br_2 to form methyl bromide, CO_2, and AgBr. This reaction is an examples of-

   (a) Wurtz reaction

   (b) Etard's reaction

   (c) Hunsdieker reaction

   (d) Perkin reaction

7. Hunsdieker reaction is used for the preparation of-

    (a) Alkyl chloride and bromides

    (b) Alkyl nitrates and nitrites

    (c) Ketenes

    (d) Alcohols

8. Lucas test is used to determine the types of

    (a) Alcohols

    (b) Acids

    (c) Amines

    (d) Carbohydrates

9. The compound which reacts most readily with Lucas reagent

    (a) CH_3CH_2Cl

    (b) $(CH_3)_2CHOH$

    (c) CH_3CH_2OH

    (d) $(CH_3)_3COH$

10. Which of the following compounds reacts slowest with Lucas reagent at room temperature.

    (a) 1-Butanol

    (b) 2-Propanol

    (c) 2-Butanol

    (d) 2-Methyl-2-propanol

11. Which alkyl halide reacts most readily by nucleophilic substitution?

    (a) CH_3CH_2Cl

    (b) CH_3CH_2I

    (c) CH_3CH_2Br

    (d) CH_3CH_3F

12. 2,2-dichloropropane reacts with aqueous KOH to give

    (a) 2,2-propane diol

    (b) Propanal

    (c) Acetone

    (d) Propene

13. Alkyl halide undergoes

    (a) Electrophilic substitution reaction

    (b) Electrophilic addition reaction

    (c) Nucleophilic substitution reaction

    (d) Nucleophilic addition reaction

14. Correct molecular formula for chloroform is

    (a) $CHCl_3$

    (b) CH_2Cl_2

    (c) CH_3Cl

    (d) CCl_4

15. Correct molecular formula for tetrachloroethylene

    (a) C_2Cl_4

    (b) $C_2H_2Cl_2$

    (c) C_2H_3Cl

    (d) C_2HCl_3

Answers for MCQs

1. (d)	2. (a)	3. (c)	4. (c)	5. (b)
6. (c)	7. (a)	8. (a)	9. (d)	10. (a)
11. (b)	12. (c)	13. (c)	14. (a)	15. (a)

Short Answer Questions

1. How can Lucas reagent be used for the distinguish of various alcohols?

2. How will one distinguish between 1-butanol and 2-butanol?

3. How can you distinguish between n-butyl alcohol and carboxylic acid?

4. What products are obtained when ethyl alcohol is treated with sulphuric acid under various conditions?

5. Bond length of C—O bond in phenol is shorter than that in methanol.

6. $(CH_3)_3C$—Br on reaction with sodium methoxide $(Na^+OCH_3^-)$ gives alkene as the main product and not an ether.

7. Discuss the reaction used for conversion of Prop-l-ene to Propan- l-ol.

8. Predict the product when ethanol is treated with Cu at 573 K,

9. Predict the product when ethyl chloride is treated with $NaOCH_3$?

10. Why do alcohols have higher boiling point as compared to ethers?

Long Answer Questions

1. Write down the strutural formulas and give IUPAC names of all isomeric alcohols of the molecular formula $CH_3CH_2CH_2CH_2CH_2OH$.

2. Give two major types of reactions of alcohols.

3. Describe the result of the oxidation of a primary alcohol.

4. Describe the result of the oxidation of a secondary alcohol.

5. Discuss the mechanism of E1 and E2 reactions of alkyl halides.

6. Discuss the mechanism of SN1 and SN2 mechanism.

7. Explain the products obtained in SN1 and SN2 mechanism.

8. What are the various evidences of E1 and E2 reactions.

Carbonyl Compounds

A carbonyl group is a functional group in which a carbon atom is doubly linked to an oxygen atom [C=O], and carbonyl compounds are compounds that include this functional group. Some of the examples of carbonyl compounds are listed in below Table.

COMPOUND	GENERAL FORMULA	STRUCTURE
ALDEHYDE	RCHO	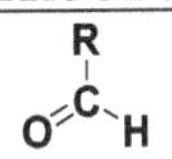
KETONE	RCOR'	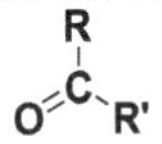
CARBOXYLIC ACID	RCOOH	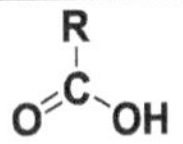
CARBOXYLATE ESTER	RCOOR'	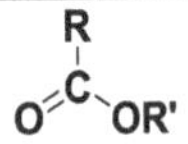
AMIDE	RCONR'R"	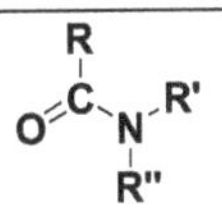
ENONE	RC(O)C(R')CR"R'''	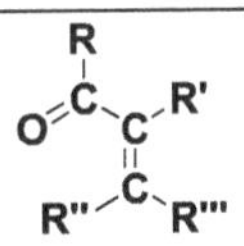
ACYL HALIDE	COX	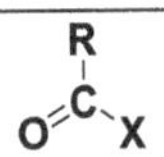
ACID ANHYDRIDE	$(RCO)_2O$	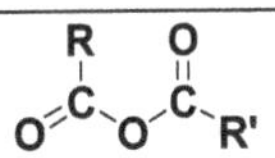
IMIDE	RC(O)N(R')C(O)R"	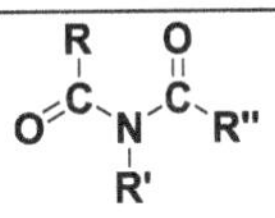

Both aldehydes and ketones show resemblance in most of their properties, although, the difference in their structure which can be seen in the form of a hydrogen atom flanked to the carbonyl group in aldehydes in place of two alkyl groups as present in ketones, give rise to some differences in their properties. This difference in properties can be seen in the form of: (i) a quicker and easy oxidation of aldehydes as compared to the ketones (ii) a greater reactivity of aldehydes towards nucleophilic addition reactions in comparison to the ketones. These compounds possess wide biological activity. Some of the biological structures having aldehyde and ketone as basic moiety are depicted in below Figure.

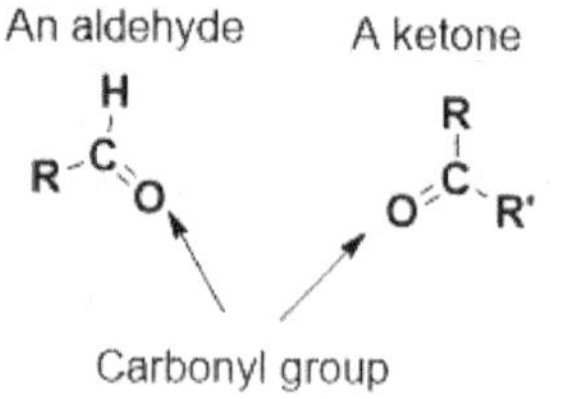

Nomenclature

The IUPAC NAMES for aldehydes:

The four steps procedure of IUPAC system common to most of the organic compounds is followed while naming aldehydes:

    (a)   Identifying and naming the parent hydrocarbon chain.

    (b)   Identifying and naming the substituents attached to parent chain.

    (c)   Assigning a locant to each substituent present in parent chain.

    (d)   Finally, the substituents are assembled alphabetically.

Aldehydes are named as alkanals by dropping terminal '-e' of the parent hydrocarbon chain and replacing it with '-al' as suffix. The longest carbon chain with aldehyde (–CHO) group is considered as the parent chain.

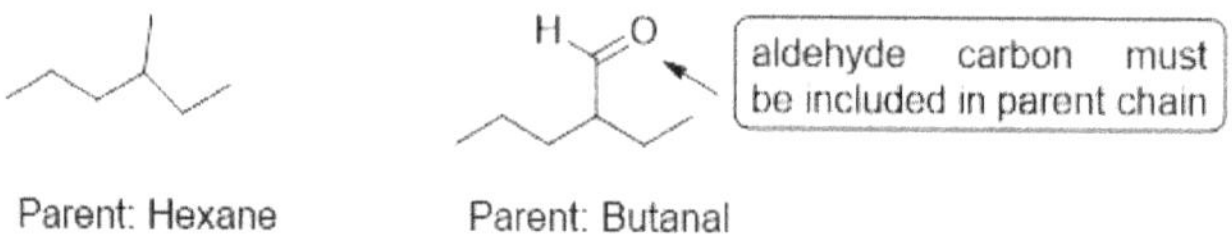

When the suffix begins with a vowel '-al' than the 'e' of alkane is dropped while when the suffix begins with a consonant '-dial' than the 'e' of alkane name is retained.

Hexanal   2-Phenyl pentanedial

The numbering of parent chain is done in such a way that number 1 is always assigned to the aldehyde carbon even if there are other substituents present like hydroxyl groups, alkyl groups or multiple bonds. Naming the position of aldehydic carbon is not necessary as it is always positioned as the number 1 carbon.

correct   incorrect

3-methylbutanal

2-ethyl-3-methylpentanal

2-chloro-3-phenylpropanal

The IUPAC NAMES for Ketones:

The ketones are named as alkanones by replacing 'e' of the parent hydrocarbon chain with the suffix 'one'.

propane   propanone

For positioning the ketone group using a locant, the IUPAC 1979 states to place the locant immediately before the parent hydrocarbon. On the other hand, the IUPAC 1993 and 2004 recommends the use of locant immediately before the suffix "-one".

3-Octanone or
Octan-3-one

Structure and Bonding

The carbonyl group consists of a double bond between carbon and oxygen. The carbon atom involved in the carbonyl group uses its two valence electrons for making a double bond with carbonyl oxygen atom. The two valence electrons of carbonyl carbon that are missing are used to create two single bonds with two additional atoms, while the remaining four electrons of carbonyl oxygen are left unshared as two lone pair electron sets. The carbonyl carbon is sp^2 hybridized and is connected to three additional atoms via three sigma bonds using its sp^2 hybrid orbitals in the carbonyl group. All of these bonds are in a plane and are about 120° apart. The 2p orbitals present on carbon and oxygen overlaps sideways to form pi-bond. The carbonyl group's oxygen atom is also sp^2 hybridized, but only one of its sp^2 orbitals participates in the creation of a sigma bond with the carbon, leaving the other two sp^2 orbitals unoccupied in the form of two sets of lone pair electrons. Large dipole moments of carbonyl compounds with dipole moments ranging from 2.3 to 2.8D show the unequal distribution of electrons in the carbonyl group. The pi electron cloud is strongly drawn towards the oxygen atom due to differences in electronegativities between carbon and oxygen (more electronegative), causing the bond to become polarized, with carbon acting as an electrophile and oxygen acting as a nucleophile.

lone pair of electrons on oxygen atom
act as hydrogen bond acceptors

The dipole moments of carbonyl compounds are higher as compared to corresponding alkenes:

$$CH_3CH_2CH{=}CH_2 \qquad CH_3CH_2CH{=}O$$

1-Butene: 0.3D   Propanal: 2.5D

Physical Properties

- Both aldehydes and ketones possess higher boiling points, due to the presence of polar carbonyl group, as compared to the non-polar compounds of similar molecular weight.

- They possess lower boiling points as compared to the corresponding alcohols and carboxylic acids due to the lack of intermolecular hydrogen bonding between two carbonyl groups, as they contain hydrogen bonded only to carbon.

- They are more soluble in water compared to alkenes due to the capability of forming hydrogen bonds with -OH groups but are less soluble than alcohols.

- Aldehydes with lower molecular weight have an unpleasant odour while higher aldehydes possess fruity smell.

- Formaldehyde is a gas with boiling point of -21° and is often used in the form of formalin (its aqueous solution) or paraformaldehyde (its solid polymer). Acetaldehyde is a gas with boiling point of 21° while aldehydes from C_3 to C_{11} are liquids and higher aldehydes exist as solids. In case of ketones, the first eleven members (C_1-C_{11}) are liquids while higher members exist as solids.

Chemical Names	B.P. (°C)	M.P. (°C)	Solubility (g/100g water)
Formaldehyde	-21	-92	Very soluble
Acetaldehyde	20	-121	infinite
Propionaldehyde	49	-81	16
n-Butyraldehyde	76	-99	7
n-Valeraldehyde	103	-91	slightly
Acetone	56	-94	Infinite
2-Pentanone	102	-78	6.3
2-Hexanone	150	-35	2.0
Acetophenone	202	21	slightly
1-Butene	-6	-185.3	Negligible
Propanol	97	-126	Miscible in all proportions

Preparations of Carbonyl Compounds

The preparation of aldehydes and ketones is done in a variety of ways. The following are a few of them:

1. **Oxidation of primary alcohols to aldehydes:** Oxidants such as potassium permanganate in alkaline solution, potassium dichromate in acidic solution, or pyridinium dichromate (PDC) or pyridinium chlorochromate (PCC) in dichloromethane or dimethyl sulfoxide in the presence of oxalyl chloride and trimethylamine are used to carry out oxidation. The aldehydes so formed can readily oxidise to corresponding carboxylic acids.

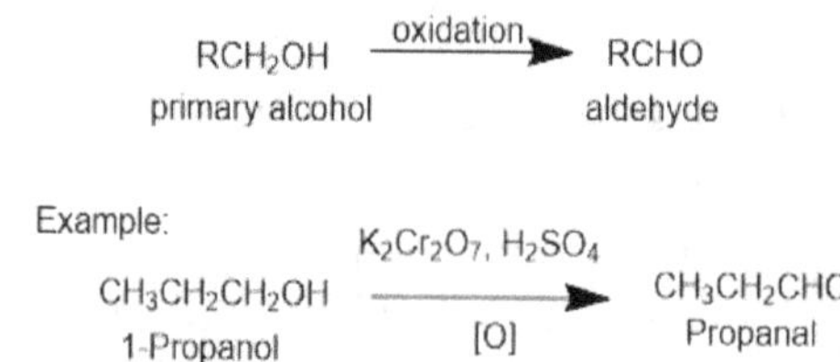

2. **Oxidation of secondary alcohols to ketones:** The secondary alcohol was further utilized to prepare corresponding ketones by spontaneous oxidation. However, ketones so obtained are not easily oxidised further.

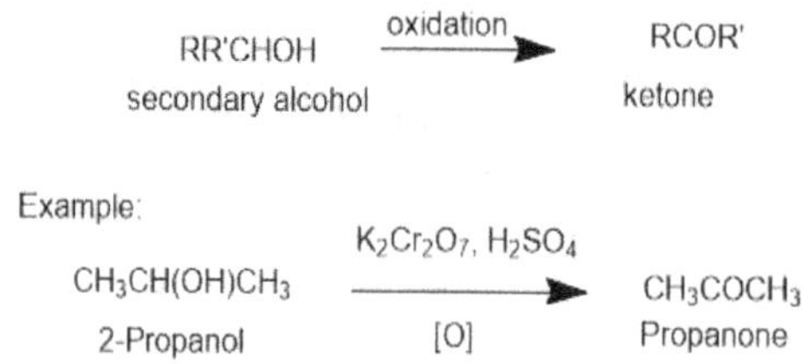

3. **Ozonolysis of alkenes:** Alkenes can be oxidised with ozone into aldehydes and ketones. The ozonide intermediate formed is hydrolysed in the presence of zinc to get the products. This method can be used for structural determination.

4. **Catalytic Dehydrogenation of alcohols:** Primary alcohols can be dehydrogenated in the presence of catalyst to aldehydes while secondary alcohols result in formation of ketones. The catalyst used can be reduced copper or silver.

Example:

$$CH_3CH(OH)CH_3 \xrightarrow[300^0]{Cu} CH_3COCH_3$$

2-Propanol   Acetone

5. **Hydration of alkynes:** Alkynes undergo hydration reaction in the presence of mixture of mercuric sulphate and sulphuric acid to give an enol intermediate as a result of markonikov addition of water to the triple bond which isomerises to aldehydes or ketones.

$$RC\equiv CR' + H_2O \xrightarrow{H_2SO_4, HgSO_4} \text{(enol intermediate)} \xrightarrow{isomerises} \text{(aldehyde or ketone)}$$

alkyne   enol intermediate   aldehyde or ketone

Examples:

$$HC\equiv CH + H_2O \xrightarrow{H_2SO_4, HgSO_4} CH_3CHO$$

acetylene   acetaldehyde

$$\text{1-Pentyne} + H_2O \xrightarrow{H_2SO_4, HgSO_4} \text{2-Pentanone}$$

1-Pentyne   2-Pentanone

6. **Friedel Crafts acylation of aromatic compounds:** Aromatic compounds undergo acylation reaction when treated with acyl chlorides or acid anhydrides in the presence of lewis acids like aluminium chloride to obtain ketones.

$$ArH + RCOCl \xrightarrow{AlCl_3} ArCOR + HCl$$

acid chloride   ketone

Example:

1-Chloro-2-phenyl ethane   Butanoyl chloride   (p-Chloroethyl)phenylpropyl ketone

7. **Hydrolysis of gem-dihalides:** The gem-dihalides can be hydrolysed to aldehydes and ketones in an alkaline solution.

$$RHCCl_2 \xrightarrow{OH^-} RHC(OH)_2 \xrightarrow{-H_2O} RCHO$$

halogen atoms attached
to terminal carbon atom   aldehyde

Example:

$$CH_3CHCl_2 \xrightarrow{OH^-} CH_3CH(OH)_2 \xrightarrow{-H_2O} CH_3CHO + H_2O$$

1,1-Dichloroethane   acetaldehyde

$$RRCCl_2 \xrightarrow{OH^-} RRC(OH)_2 \xrightarrow{-H_2O} RCOR$$

halogen atoms attached
to any carbon other than
theterminal carbon atom   ketone

Example:

$$CH_3C(Cl_2)CH_3 \xrightarrow{2\ OH^-} CH_3C(OH)_2CH_3 \xrightarrow{-H_2O} CH_3COCH_3 + H_2O$$

2,2-Dichloroethane   acetaldehyde

8. **Reduction of esters:** Esters undergo reduction in the presence of diisobutylaluminium hydride to form aldehydes.

ester $\xrightarrow[\text{2. }H_2O]{\text{1. DIBAL-H}}$ RCHO (aldehyde)

Example:

$$CH_3COOC_2H_5 \xrightarrow[\text{2. }H_2O]{\text{1. DIBAL-H}} CH_3CHO$$

ethyl acetate   acetaldehyde

9. **Decomposition of carboxylic acids:** Carboxylic acids when passed over heated manganese oxide or thorium oxide give ketones.

$$2RCOOH \xrightarrow{MnO,\ 300^0} RCOR + CO_2 + H_2O$$

acid   ketone

(other then formic acid)

Example:

$$2CH_3COOH \xrightarrow{MnO,\ 300^0} CH_3COCH_3 + CO_2 + H_2O$$

acetic acid   acetone

10. **Reactions of acids and organometallic reagents:** Organometallic reagents like phenyl lithium can react with acids to give carbonyl compounds.

11. **Reduction of nitriles:** Nitriles on reduction with reducing agents like lithium triethoxy aluminium hydride or stannous chloride in hydrochloride solution in ether and further hydrolysis yield aldehydes.

$$RCN \xrightarrow[\text{ether}]{SnCl_2\text{-HCl}} RHC{=}NH.HCl \xrightarrow{\text{hydrolysis}} RCHO + NH_4Cl$$

                                   aldimine hydrochloride

Example:

Chemical Reactions of Carbonyl Compounds

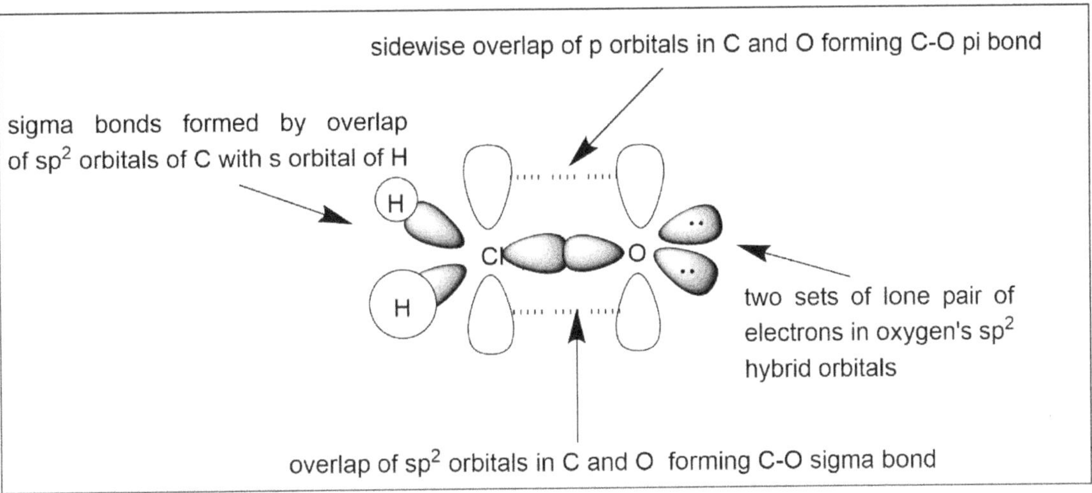

As discussed above, the polarization in the carbonyl group due to higher electronegativity of oxygen render the carbon atom relatively electron deficient therefore acting as an electrophile while the oxygen atom behaves as a nucleophile making the carbonyl group highly reactive. The electrophilic nature of the carbon atom can also be explained as follows:

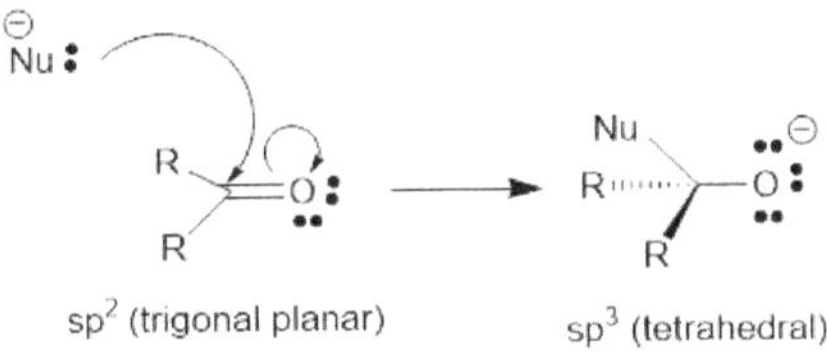

Both the resonance and inductive effects give the carbon atom a tiny positive charge, making it electron-deficient and vulnerable to nucleophilic assault. After being attacked by a nucleophile, the sp^2 hybridized carbon atom converts to sp3 hybridization.

Also, aldehydes show greater reactivity towards nucleophilic attack as compared to ketones which is attributed to steric and electronic effects.

(a) Steric effects: In case of ketones, there are two alkyl groups (electron donors) present one on both sides of the carbonyl group resulting in greater steric interactions and lesser reactivity when a nucleophile approach it as compared to the aldehydes where only one alkyl group is attached to carbonyl group.

(b) Electronic effects: Due to the electron donating nature of alkyl groups, the δ^+ charge on the carbonyl carbon is less stabilised in transition state. In case of ketones possessing two alkyl groups around carbonyl group while it is more stabilised in aldehydes. Therefore, aldehydes show greater reactivity towards nucleophilic attack than the ketones.

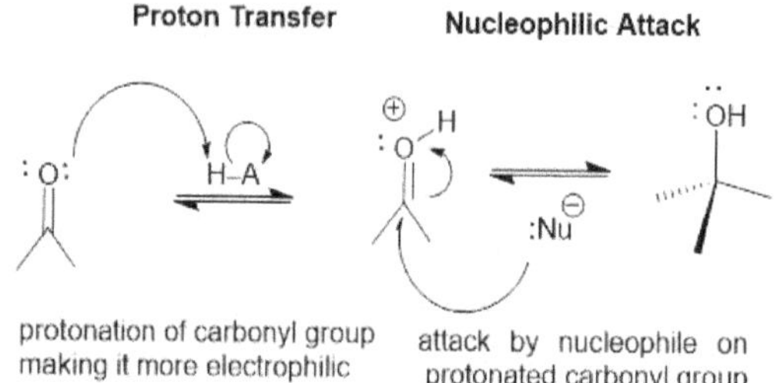

ketone with two alkyl groups (electron donors) stabilizing the partial positive charge

aldehyde with one alkyl group (electron donor) stabilizing the partial positive charge

Nucleophilic Addition Reactions

Acid-catalysed mechanism: In acidic conditions, the first step includes the protonation of the carbonyl group by an acid which renders it even more electrophilic which is basically of value in case of weaker nucleophiles like water or alcohols.

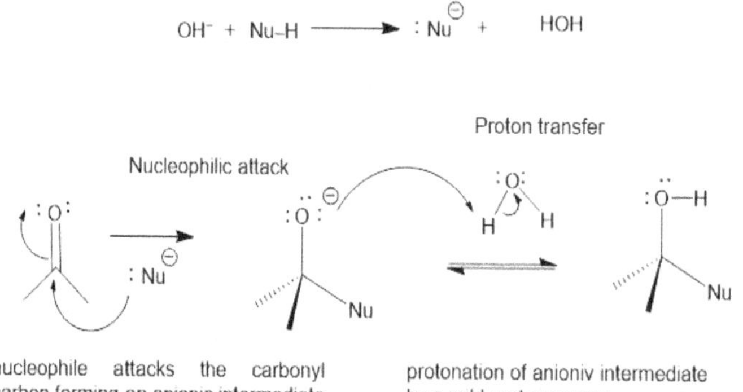

Base-catalysed mechanism: In basic conditions, the base first liberates the nucleophile from its conjugate acid, which then attacks the electrophilic carbonyl carbon.

generation of nucleophile

OH⁻ + Nu–H ⟶ :Nu⁻ + HOH

Nucleophilic attack

Proton transfer

:Nu⁻

:O–H

Nu

nucleophile attacks the carbonyl carbon forming an anionic intermediate

protonation of anioniv intermediate by a mild proton source

Some orbital considerations: In nucleophilic addition reactions, as the nucleophile approaches the carbonyl group, the electrons from its HOMO start moving towards the LUMO (π^* antibonding) of carbonyl group. Therefore, whenever the coefficient of this LUMO carbonyl carbon is larger which means the carbonyl group is more polarized than in that case the HOMO-LUMO interaction is higher. With the movement of electrons to the π^* orbital of carbon, the π bond between carbon and oxygen began to break while these π electrons migrates towards the electronegative oxygen atom giving it a negative charge. This whole process results in breaking of a π bond while simultaneously a new σ bond is formed and also this result in the generation of a tetrahedral sp³ carbon atom from the earlier triagonal planar sp² hybridized carbonyl carbon atom.

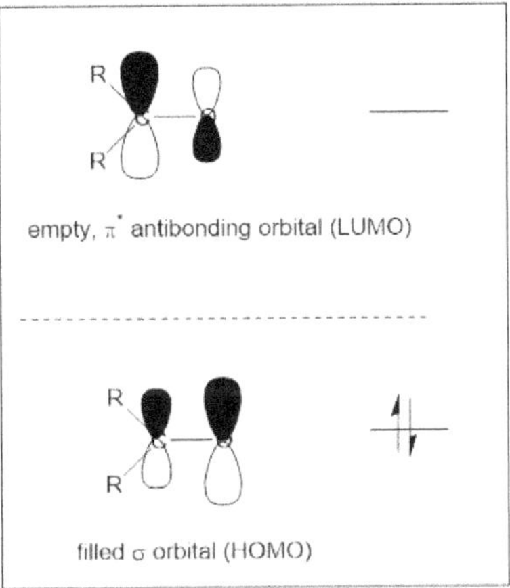

Hemiacetals and Acetals Formation

Aldehydes and ketones undergo nucleophilic addition reaction with alcohols which leads to the formation of a hemiacetal, characterised by the presence of hydroxyl and alkoxy group on the carbon atom.

Mechanism:

1. Acid catalysed:

2. Base catalysed:

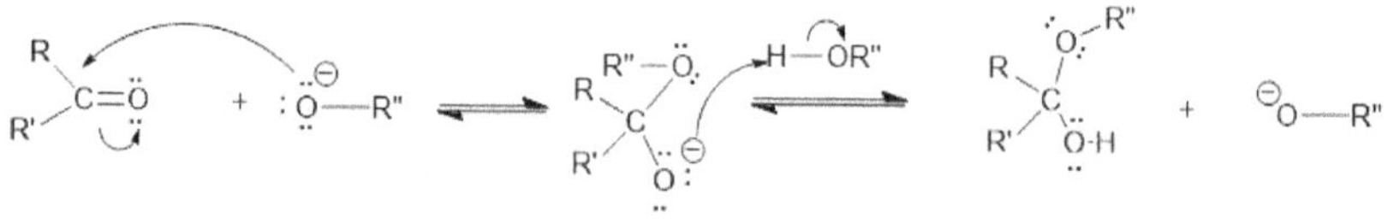

nucleophilic   alkoxide   anion   attacks   hemiacetal
the carbonyl carbon atom forming a new alkoxide anion

Hemiacetal forms above can further react with another mole of alcohol to give an acetal, characterised by the presence of two -OR groups in same carbon atom.

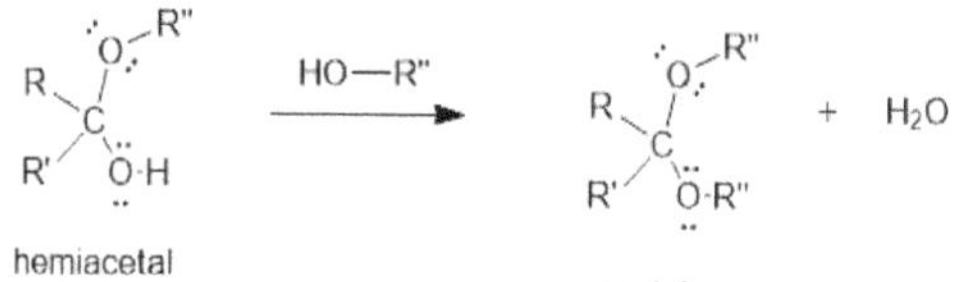

hemiacetal
(unstable to isolate)

acetal
(stable)

Mechanism: Acid catalysed

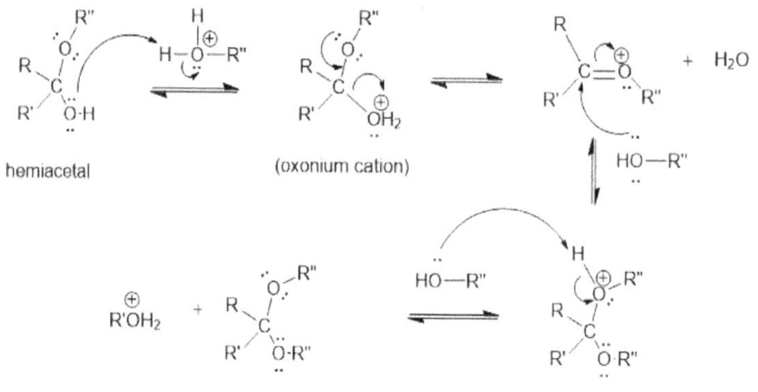

hemiacetal

(oxonium cation)

acetal

Formation of Bisulfite Addition Compound

The non-bonded electrons present on the nucleophilic bisulfite attacks the electrophilic carbonyl carbon of aldehyde or ketone giving a positive charge to the sulphur atom followed by a proton transfer to the negatively charged oxygen atom leading to the formation of final product, the bisulfite addition compound. This reaction can be used for purification of liquid aldehydes by recrystallization.

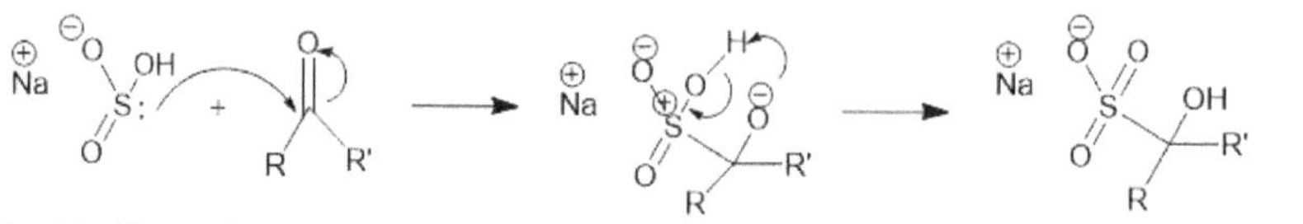

sodium bisulfite   aldehyde or ketone

bisulfite addition compound

Addition of Water (Hydration)

Acid or base catalyses the hydration of aldehydes or ketones leading to formation of 1,1-diols or geminal diols. The reaction is reversible and is favoured towards the gem-diol in case of simpler aldehydes while for sterically hindered carbonyl compounds, equilibrium is shifted towards the left.

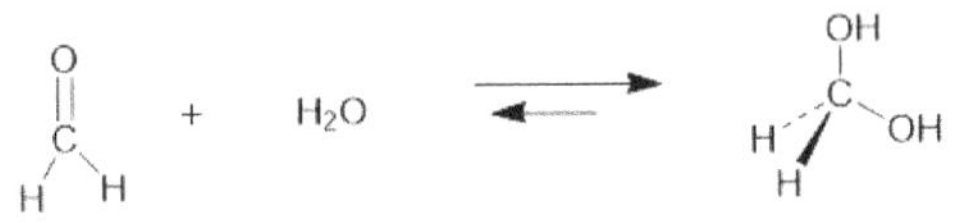

formaldehyde (0.1%)

formaldehyde hydrate, a gem diol (99.9%)

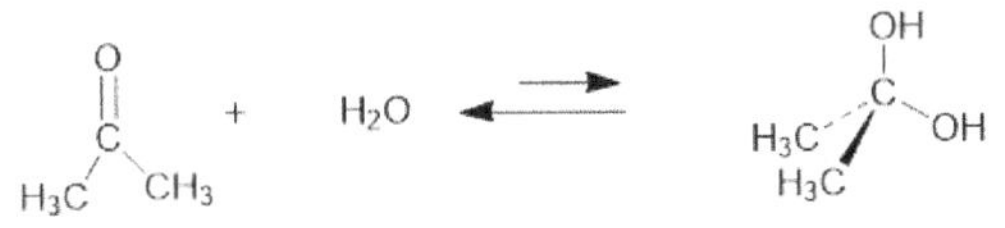

acetone (99.9%)

acetone hydrate, a gem diol (0.1%)

Mechanism:

1. Acid catalysed:

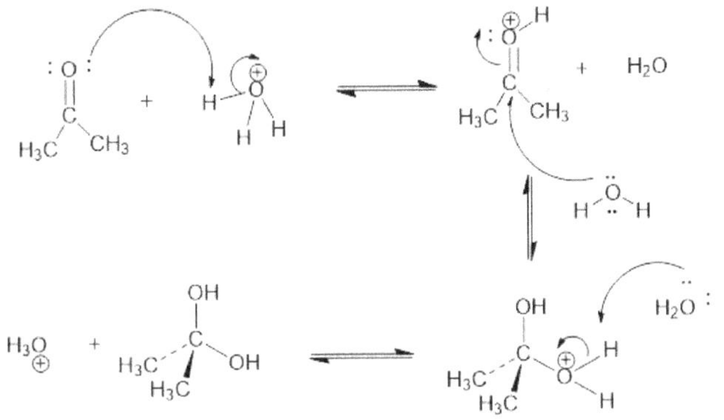

hydrate (gem diol)

2. Base catalysed:

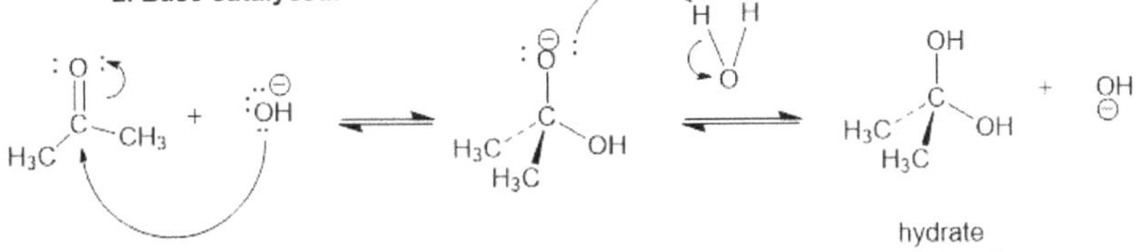

hydrate (gem diol)

Addition of Grignard Reagent

Grignard reagents produce alcohols through a nucleophilic addition reaction with aldehydes and ketones. Due to electronegativity difference between carbon (2.5) and magnesium (1.2), the bond between them is polar. Grignard reagents act as good nucleophiles and create tetrahedral carbonyl addition compounds with aldehydes and ketones as a result.

1. Addition of formaldehyde:

$$CH_3CH_2MgBr \ + \ HCHO \ \xrightarrow{\text{ether}} \ CH_3CH_2-CH_2 \xrightarrow[H_2O]{HCl} CH_3CH_2-CH_2 \ + \ Mg^{2+}$$

grignard reagent   formaldehyde   magnesium alkoxide   1-Propanol (a primary alcohol)

2. Addition of a higher aldehyde:

$$+ \ CH_3CHO \xrightarrow{\text{ether}} \ \xrightarrow[H_2O]{HCl} \ + \ Mg^{2+}$$

acetaldehyde   1-Cyclohexylethanol (secondary alcohol)

3. Addition of ketones:

$$\xrightarrow{\text{ether}} \ \xrightarrow[H_2O]{HCl} \ + \ Mg^{2+}$$

acetone   2-Phenyl-2-propanol (tertiary alcohol)

Addition of Organometallic Reagents

In organolithium compounds, the metal atoms are electropositive thereby making the C-metal bond polarized. As a result, these organometallic compounds behave as strong nucleophiles forming addition compounds with aldehydes and ketones.

$$Me\text{-}Li \ + \ RCHO \xrightarrow[\text{2. }H_2O]{\text{1. THF}}$$

organometalic compound   aldehyde   an alcohol

Mechanism:

$$Me\text{-}Li \ + \ \longrightarrow \ \longrightarrow$$

Addition of Amines

Primary amines undergo nucleophilic addition reaction with aldehydes and ketones to give imines while secondary amines yield enamines.

Wittig Reaction: Addition of Phosphorous Ylides

The triphenyl phosphorous ylide (phosphorane) show nucleophilic addition to aldehydes and ketones yielding an unstable oxaphosphetane intermediate which spontaneously decompose to give an alkene.

Addition of Hydrogen Cyanide

HCN show nucleophilic addition reaction with aldehydes and ketones resulting in the formation of cyanohydrins, tetrahedral carbonyl addition compounds.

RCHO + HCN ⇌ R–C(OH)(H)–CN

aldehyde or ketone

a cyanohydrine

Mechanism:

Formation of Thioacetals

Thioacetals are formed by nucleophilic addition of thiols to aldehydes and ketones.

aldehyde or ketone   methanethiol   a thioacetal

a ketone   a thiol   a thioacetal

H_2 | Raney   nickle
(desulfurization)

Aldol Condensation

Two molecules of an aldehyde or a ketone can undergo self-addition reaction in a reversible manner in the presence of a base to give a product which possess both an aldehyde and an alcohol and so called an aldol (a β-hydroxy carbonyl compound).

two molecules of an aldehyde   an aldol (a β hydroxy carbonyl compound)

The resultant aldol is isolable, but it can also undergo condensation with the loss of a water molecule, forming a conjugated,-unsaturated carbonyl chemical. Aldol condensation is the name for this entire reaction.

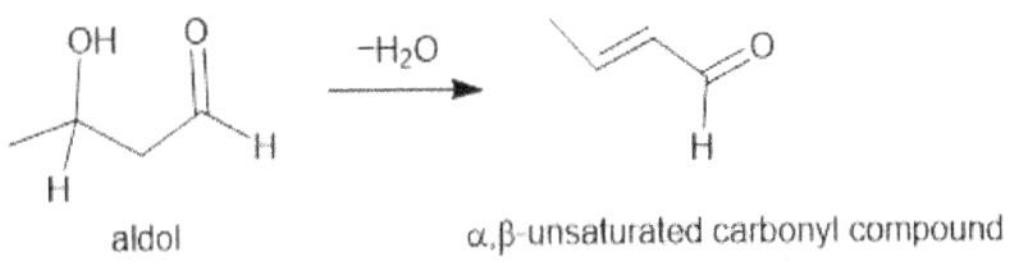

The presence of at least one -hydrogen atom in aldehydes is required for aldol condensation to occur; otherwise, the reaction will not take place.

Mechanism

1) **Proton abstraction:** Base abstracts proton from the β-carbon atom of the aldehyde, esulting in the creation of a carbanion ion (an enolate anion).

2) **Alkoxide anion formation:** The nucleophilic enolate ion reacts at the electrophilic carbonyl carbon of another aldehyde to form an alkoxide ion.

3) **Aldol formation:** The alkoxide anion absorbs a proton from the solvent, water, and produces aldol as a result.

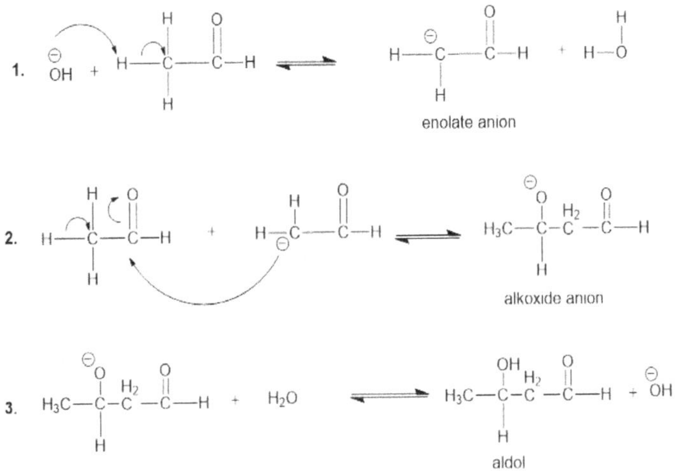

Dehydration of aldols: Aldols on heating in the presence of a base or in acidic medium may undergo dehydration resulting in the formation of α, β-unsaturated carbonyl compound.

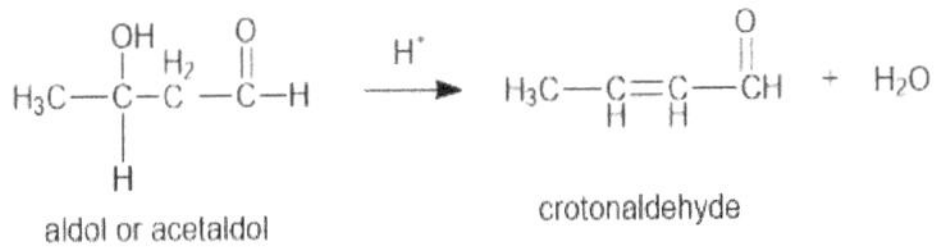

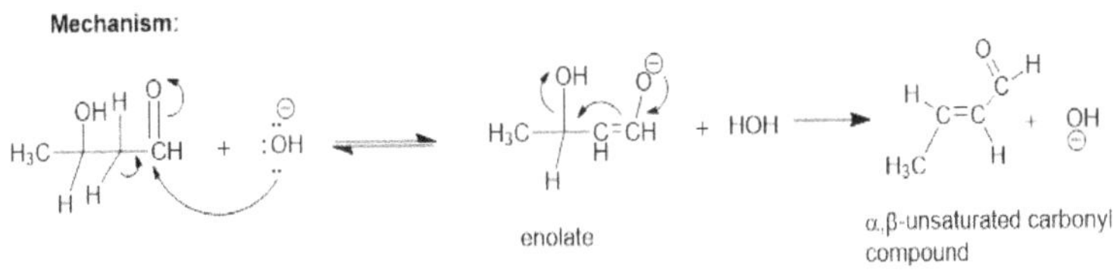

Aldol Condensation in ketones: Ketones undergo aldol condensation to a lesser extent as compared to aldehydes due to the steric hinderance on carbonyl group by two alkyl groups.

$$2\ CH_3COCH_3 \xrightarrow{\ ^{\ominus}OH\ } H_3C-\underset{CH_3}{\overset{OH}{C}}-CH_2-CO-CH_3 \xrightarrow{\ ^{\oplus}H\ } H_3C-CH=C(CH_3)-CO-CH_3$$

acetone   diacetone alcohol (aldol)   mesityl oxide

Crossed Aldol Condensation: It is a condensation reaction in which two different aldehydes and/or ketones (each possessing α hydrogen atoms) undergo condensation in the presence of a base to give mixture of four aldol products.

$$CH_3CHO\ +\ RCH_2CHO \xrightarrow{\ ^{\ominus}OH\ } CH_3CH(OH)CHRCHO$$
crossed aldol

$$RCH_2CHO\ +\ CH_3CHO \xrightarrow{\ ^{\ominus}OH\ } RCH_2CH(OH)CH_2CHO$$
crossed aldol

$$CH_3CHO\ +\ CH_3CHO \xrightarrow{\ ^{\ominus}OH\ } CH_3CH(OH)CH_2CHO$$
simple aldol

$$RCH_2CHO\ +\ RCH_2CHO \xrightarrow{\ ^{\ominus}OH\ } RCH_2CH(OH)CHRCHO$$
simple aldol

Cannizzaro Reaction

It is a redox reaction between two molecules of aldehydes (lacking α hydrogen) in the presence of a base to yield a molecule of alcohol and carboxylic acid. This reaction involves oxidation of one molecule of an aldehyde with simultaneous reduction of the other molecule. Usually, the aldehyde is kept at room temperature with alkali hydroxide to yield the product. Under the reaction conditions, the aldehydes bearing α hydrogen have the tendency to undergo aldol condensation.

$$2\ RCHO \xrightarrow{\ base\ } RCH_2OH\ +\ RCOOH$$

aldehyde   primary alcohol   carboxylic acid
(lacking α hydrogen)

Mechanism:

carboxylic acid   primary alcohol

Crossed Cannizzaro Reaction

The redox reaction between two different aldehydes (lacking α hydrogen) like formaldehyde and benzaldehyde in the presence of a base to give an alcohol and a carboxylic acid as a product is termed as crossed cannizzaro reaction.

benzaldehyde   formaldehyde   benzylalcohol   formic acid

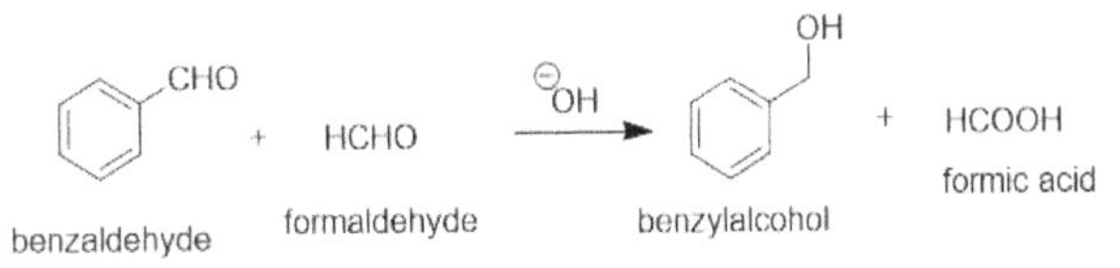

Perkin Condensation

Perkin condensation is the condensation of an aromatic aldehyde with an acid anhydride in the presence of a base, such as alkali salts of acids, to form α-β unsaturated aromatic acids.

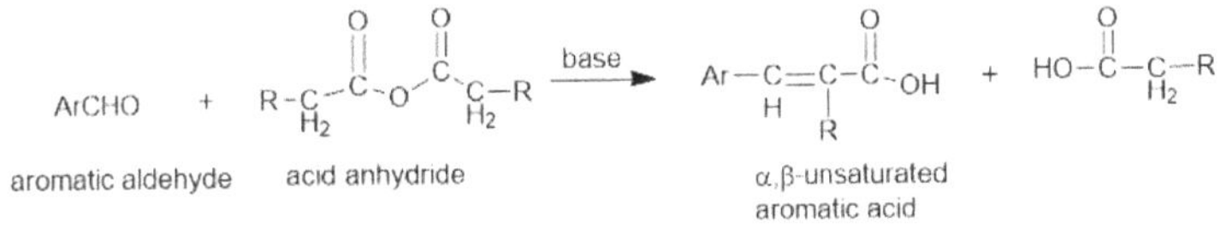

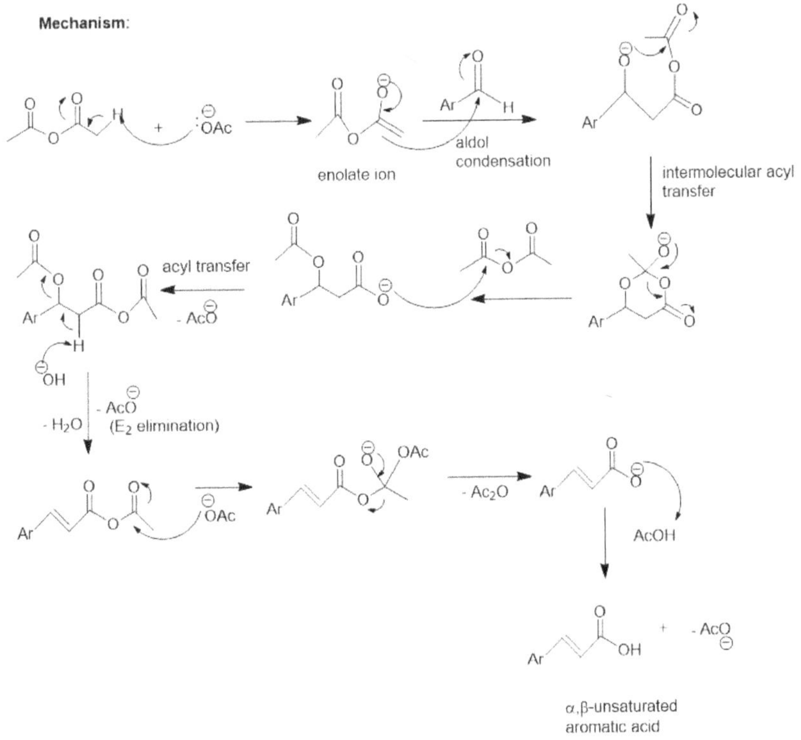

aromatic aldehyde   acid anhydride α,β-unsaturated
                                                    aromatic acid

Mechanism:

enolate ion

aldol condensation

intermolecular acyl transfer

acyl transfer

$-$ H₂O   (E₂ elimination)

AcOH

α,β-unsaturated
aromatic acid

Benzoin Condensation

The addition reaction between two aldehydes usually aromatic aldehydes or glyoxals to yield α-hydroxy ketones is termed as benzoin condensation.

Benzaldehyde

Benzoin
(α-hydroxyketone)

Mechanism:

Benzoin
(α-hydroxyketone)

Qualitative Test

1. **Oxidation:** Aldehydes can easily undergo oxidation even in the presence of mild oxidising reagents to give corresponding carboxylic acids while ketones can't. This is basically due to the difference in their structures as aldehydes possess a hydrogen atom which is easily abstracted during oxidation while in case of ketones abstraction of alkyl or aryl groups is difficult.

$$RCHO \xrightarrow{\text{oxidise}} RCOOH$$

aldehyde   carboxylic acid

furfural   furoic acid

Mechanism:

aldehyde   chromic acid   chromate ester   carboxylic acid

Tollen's Test (Silver Mirror test):

Tollen's reagent is an aqueous solution of silver nitrate, ammonia and sodium hydroxide which contains diaminosilver(I) ions which has the potential to oxidise aldehyde into carboxylate anions while simultaneously silver is reduced to metallic silver which can be seen in the form of silver mirror along the walls of the test tube.

$$RCHO \xrightarrow[H_2O]{Ag(NH_3)_2^{\oplus}} RCOO^{\ominus} + Ag\downarrow$$

aldehyde   carboxylate anion   silver mirror

cyclohexanone
(keto form)   cyclohexanone
(enol form)   hexanedioic acid

Ketones undergo oxidation only under special conditions or with strong oxidising agents.

cyclohexanone
(keto form)   cyclohexanone
(enol form)   hexanedioic acid

2. **Reduction:** Aldehydes on reduction with reducing agents like lithium aluminium hydride or metal catalysts converts to primary alcohol while ketones get reduced to secondary alcohols.

cinnamaldehyde   cinnamyl alcohol
(primary alcohol)

cyclopentanone   cyclopentanol
(secondary alcohol)

Mechanism:

sodium borohydride ketone tetrahedral carbonyl addition compound secondary alcohol

3. Schiff test: It is a detection test for aldehydes which when treated with Schiff reagent (colourless), give a characteristic magenta colour. The Schiff reagent is obtained in the form of a reaction product of a dye formulation like fuchsin and sodium bisulfite.

decolorized schiff reagent + RCHO $\longrightarrow$ magenta color complex

aldehyde

4. Reaction with ammonia derivatives:

Some ammonia derivatives containing a primary amine group show addition reaction with carbonyl groups forming unstable intermediates which undergo elimination of a water molecule yielding addition products possessing carbon- nitrogen double bond. These reactions are used as qualitative tests for identification of aldehydes and ketones.

hydroxylamine oxime

phenylhydrazine phenylhydrazone

semicarbazide semicarbazone

Structure and Uses

The basic structural features of aldehyde and ketones make its importance in pharmaceutical and chemical industry for variety of uses from house hold to translational research. Some of the shortlisted biological compounds prepared from aldehydes and ketones are listed in below Table.

S. NO.	COMPOUNDS	STRUCTURE	USES
1	FORMALDEHYDE	$H-\overset{H}{\underset{}{C}}=O$	• Its vapours are used as disinfectant • Formalin is used as preservative for biological specimens • Formalin is used for tanning • In production of plastics like Bakelite
2	PARALDEHYDE		• A CNS depressant • Used as anticonvulsant, hypnotic, sedative • Used in cough medicines
3	ACETONE	$H_3C-\overset{CH_3}{\underset{}{C}}=O$	• Used as an organic solvent • As acetylene carrier • As a cleanser in laboratories • Solvent in pharmaceutical industry • Denaturant in denatured alcohol
4	CHLORAL HYDRATE		• As sedative and hypnotic • In organic synthesis • As an ingredient in Hoyer's solution, melzer's reagent
5	HEXAMINE		• In preparation of phenolic resins • As mandelic acid salt, used in urinary tract infections • To treat sweating and odor • As staining agent in histology • As food additive • In organic synthesis
6	BENZALDEHYDE		• To impart almond flavour in food and scents • As precursor in organic synthesis • As a bee repellent
7	VANILIN		• As a flavouring agent in sweet foods, icecream and chockolate industries, baked foods • In perfumes • In medicines to mask unpleasant odor • As a visualizing stain in TLC
8	CINNAMALDEHYDE		• As a flavouring agent in icecreams, candies, beverages • In perfumes • As insecticide • As corrosion inhibitor for ferrous alloys

MCQs

1. Alkyl halide undergoes

    (a) Electrophilic substitution reaction

    (b) Electrophilic addition reaction

    (c) Nucleophilic substitution reaction

    (d) Nucleophilic addition reaction

1. The correct sequence of steps involved in the mechanism of cannizaro's reaction is:

    (a) Nucleophilic attack, transfer of H^- and transfer of H^+

    (b) Electrophilic attack by OH^-, transfer of H^+ and transfer of H^-

    (c) Transfer of H-, transfer of H^+ and nucleophilic attack

    (d) Transfer of H^+, nucleophilic attack and transfer of H^-

2. Benzaldehyde and acetone can be best distinguished using:

    (a) Hydrazine   (b) Tollen's test

    (b) Sodium hydroxide   (d) 2,4-DNP

3. In the following sequence of reactions, the alkene affords the compound B,

$$H_3C-\overset{H}{\underset{H}{C}}=\underset{}{C}-CH_3 \xrightarrow{O_3} A \xrightarrow[Zn]{H_2O} B$$

    The compound B is:-

    (a) CH_3COCH_3 (b) CH_3CH_2CHO

    (c) CH_3CHO (d) $CH_3CH_2COCH_3$

4. A mixture of benzaldehyde and formaldehyde on heating with aqueous NaOH solution gives:-

    (a) Benzyl alcohol and sodium formate

    (b) Sodium benzoate and methyl alcohol

    (c) Sodium benzoate and sodium formate

    (d) Benzyl alcohol and methyl alcohol

5. Which of the following has most acidic hydrogen

    (a) 3-Hexanone   (b) 2,4-Hexanedione

    (c) 2,5-Hexanedione   (d) 2,3-Hexadione

6. The carbon atom of a carbonyl group is

    (a) sp hybridised   (b) sp^2 hybridised

    (c) sp^3 hybridised   (d) none of these

7. Acetone reacts with HCN to form a cyanohydrin. It is an example of

    (a) Electrophilic addition
    (b) Electrophilic substitution recation
    (c) Nucleophilic addition
    (d) Nucleophilic substitution

8. Which of the following reagents will react readily with both aldehydes and ketones?

    (a) Grignard reagent
    (b) Fehling's reagent
    (c) Tollen's reagent
    (d) Schiff's reagent

9. Boiling acetaldehyde (CH_3CHO) reacts with chlorine gas to give:

    a)   [structure: H_3C—C(=O)—Cl]
    b)   [structure: Cl_3C—C(=O)—H]

    c) CH_3CHCl_2
    d) $CHCl_3$

10. The reaction of ethanal with one equivalent of methanol and a trace of an acid will give

    (a) Acetal
    (b) Hemiacetal
    (c) Ketal
    (d) Hemiketal

11. Rosenmund reduction used for conversion of acid chloride to aldehydes in the presence of:

    (a) $Pd/BaSO_4$ (Poisoned)
    (b) Zn/HCl
    (c) MnO
    (d) $[Co(CO)_4]_2$

12. Fehling's solution used for the detection of aldehyde where deep blue colour changes to brick red. Brick red is due to the formation of:

    (a) $CuSO_4$
    (b) CuO
    (c) Cu_2O
    (d) $AgNO_3$

13. Low molecular weight aldehydes and ketones show appreciable boiling point. Choose the correct reason:

    (a) The ability of the molecule to form strong H bonds
    (b) Carbonyl oxygen form H bond with other carbonyl
    (c) Polar carbonyl group attract other polar molecules
    (d) Carbonyl group to attract other electrophile and form bonds

14. Cyclopentanol on oxidation give:

    (a) Cyclopentene
    (b) Cyclopentanone
    (c) Cyclopentane
    (d) Cyclopentanal

15. Choose the incorrect statements:

    (a) Aldol is syrupy liquid β-hydroxy aldehyde or β-hydroxy ketone

(b) Aldol on heating eliminates water by E1cB mechanism

(c) On heating it gives back aldehyde and ketone

(d) On heating it give α,β-unsaturated aldehyde and α,β-unsaturated ketone

Answers for MCQs

1. (a)	2. (b)	3. (c)	4. (a)	5. (b)
6. (b)	7. (c)	8. (a)	9. (b)	10. (b)
11. (a)	12. (c)	13. (d)	14. (b)	15. (c)

Short Question Answers

1. What is Tollen's reagent? Write one usefulness of this reagent.

2. Arrange the following compounds in an increasing order of their reactivity in nucleophilic addition reactions: ethanal, propanal, propanone, butanone.

3. Give a chemical test to distinguish between Ethanal and Propanal.

4. Give a chemical test to distinguish between Propanal and Propanone.

5. Formaldehyde does not take part in Aldol condensation. Why ?

6. Give the structure and IUPAC name of the product formed when propanone is reacted with methylmagnesium bromide followed by hydrolysis.

7. Rearrange the following compounds in the increasing order of their boiling points: (All India 2013)

    CH_3 — CHO, CH_3 — CH_2 — OH, CH_3 — CH_2— CH_3

8. Ethanal is soluble in water. Why?

9. What type of aldehydes undergo Cannizaro reaction?

10. Arrange the following compound groups in the increasing order of their property indicated: Propanol, Propane, Propanal (boiling point)

11. Write the reactions involved in the following reactions:
     (i) Clemmensen reduction
     (ii) Cannizzaro reaction

12. Write down test to distinguish between aldehydes and ketones.

13. What do you mean by Haloform test of ketones.

14. Do the following conversions in not more than two steps:
     (i) Benzoic acid to benzaldehyde
     (ii) Ethyl benzene to Benzoic acid
     (iii) Propanone to Propene

15. Illustrate the following name reactions by giving example:
    (i) Cannizzaro's reaction
    (ii) Clemmensen reduction

    (b) An organic compound A contains 69.77% carbon, 11.63% hydrogen and rest oxygen. The molecular mass of the compound is 86. It does not reduce Tollen's reagent but forms an addition compound with sodium hydrogen sulphite and gives positive iodoform test. On vigorous oxidation it gives ethanoic and propanoic acids. Derive the possible structure of compound A.

16. Explain the mechanism of a nucleophilic attack on the carbonyl group of an aldehyde or a ketone.
    (b) An organic compound (A) (molecular formula $C_9H_{16}O_2$) was hydrolysed with dilute sulphuric acid to give a carboxylic acid (B) and an alcohol (C). Oxidation of (C) with chromic acid also produced (B). On dehydration (C) gives but-1-ene. Write the equations for the reactions involved

17. Arrange the following in the increasing order of their boiling points:
    (i) $CH_3CH_2CH_2CHO$, $CH_3CH_2CH_2CH_2OH$, $H_5C_2-O-C_2H_5$, $CH_3CH_2CH_2CH_2CH_3$
    (ii) CH_3CHO, CH_3CH_2OH, CH_3OCH_3, $CH_3CH_2CH_3$

18. What happens when formaldehyde is treated with dilute sodium hydroxide?

19. Predict the product when acetone is treated with barium hydroxide.

Long Question Answers

1. What product will be formed on reaction of propanal with 2-methylpropanal in the presence of NaOH? What products will be formed? Write the name of the reaction also.

2. Compound 'A' was prepared by oxidation of compound 'B' with alkaline KMnO4. Compound 'A' on reduction with lithium aluminium hydride gets converted back to compound 'B'. When compound 'A' is heated with compound B in the presence of H_2SO_4 it produces fruity smell of compound C to which family the compounds 'A', 'B' and 'C' belong to?

3. An alkene 'A' (Mol. formula C_5H_{10}) on ozonolysis gives a mixture of two compounds 'B' and 'C'. Compound 'B' gives positive Fehling's test and also forms iodoform on treatment with I_2 and NaOH. Compound 'C' does not give Fehling's test but forms iodoform. Identify the compounds A, B and C. Write the reaction for ozonolysis and formation of iodoform from B and C.

4. An aromatic compound 'A' (Molecular formula C_8H_8O) gives positive 2, 4-DNP test. It gives a yellow precipitate of compound 'B' on treatment with iodine and sodium hydroxide solution. Compound 'A' does not give Tollen's or Fehling's test. On drastic oxidation with potassium permanganate it forms a carboxylic acid 'C' (Molecular formula $C_7H_6O_2$), which is also formed along with the yellow compound in the above reaction. Identify A, B and C and write all the reactions involved.

5. Write down functional isomers of a carbonyl compound with molecular formula C_3H_6O. Which isomer will react faster with HCN and why? Explain the mechanism of the reaction also. Will the reaction lead to the completion with the conversion of whole reactant into product at reaction conditions? If a strong acid is added to the reaction mixture what will be the effect on concentration of the product and why?

6. When liquid 'A' is treated with a freshly prepared ammoniacal silver nitrate solution, it gives bright silver mirror. The liquid forms a white crystalline solid on treatment with sodium hydrogensulphite. Liquid 'B' also forms a white crystalline solid with sodium hydrogensulphite but it does not give test with ammoniacal silver nitrate. Which of the two liquids is aldehyde? Write the chemical equations of these reactions also.

7. An organic compound (A) with molecular formula C_8H_8O forms an orange-red precipitate with 2,4-DNP reagent and gives yellow precipitate on heating with iodine in the presence of sodium hydroxide. It neither reduces Tollens' or Fehlings' reagent nor does it decolourise bromine water or Baeyer's reagent. On drastic oxidation with chromic acid, it gives a carboxylic acid (B) having molecular formula $C_7H_6O_2$. Identify the compounds (A) and (B) and explain the reactions involved.

8. Give general mechanism of nucleophilic addition reactions of carbonyl compounds.

9. Write a short note on Wittig reaction.

10. Discuss methods of preparation of aldehydes and ketones.

11. Discuss in detail qualitative test used for the identification of aldehydes and ketones.

12. What is Cannizaro's reaction and discuss the conditions necessary for the molecule to exhibit Cannizaro reaction.

13. Write down the various chemical reactions of aldehydes and ketones.

14. Explain in detail the structure of carbonyl compounds and also tell why carbonyl compounds undergo nucleophilic addition reactions.

Unit - 5

Carboxylic Acids and Amines

Carboxylic Acids

Organic substances with one or more carboxyl groups, -COOH, in their molecules are known as carboxylic acids. The term carboxyl comes from combining the terms carbonyl (-C=O) and hydroxyl group (-OH).

According to the amount of carboxyl groups contained in the molecule, carboxylic acids are categorised as mono-, di-, or tri- carboxylic acids.

$$H-\overset{\overset{\displaystyle O}{\|}}{C}-OH \qquad \text{Formic Acid}$$

$$CH_3COOH \qquad \text{Acetic Acid}$$

$$CH_3CH_2COOH \qquad \text{Propanoic Acid}$$

Monocarboxylic Acids

$$\begin{array}{l} COOH \\ | \\ COOH \end{array} \qquad \text{Oxalic Acid}$$

$$H_2C \overset{\displaystyle COOH}{\underset{\displaystyle COOH}{<}} \qquad \text{Malonic Acid}$$

$$\begin{array}{l} H_2C-COOH \\ | \\ H_2C-COOH \end{array} \qquad \text{Succinic Acid}$$

Dicarboxylic Acids

Structure and Acidic Character of Carboxylic Acids

The contributing structures of carboxylic structure are as follows and the carboxyl group is resonance hybrid of both the contributing structures:

131

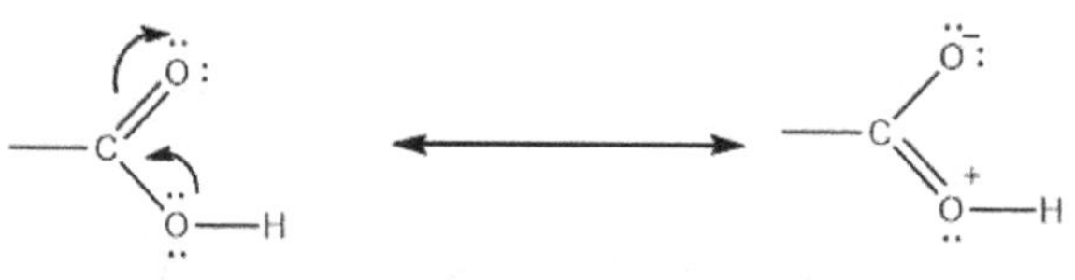

(I)   (II)

Structure (II) involves charge separation hence, it is less stable and make lesser contribution towards resonance hybrid. Whereas structure (I) is more stable and makes major contribution towards resonance hybrid.

In structure (II) it can be observed that there is separation of charge and oxygen atom bears positive charge. Due to positive charge on oxygen, release of proton from oxygen becomes very easy and hence carboxylic acids release H^+ (proton) and forms carboxylate ion.

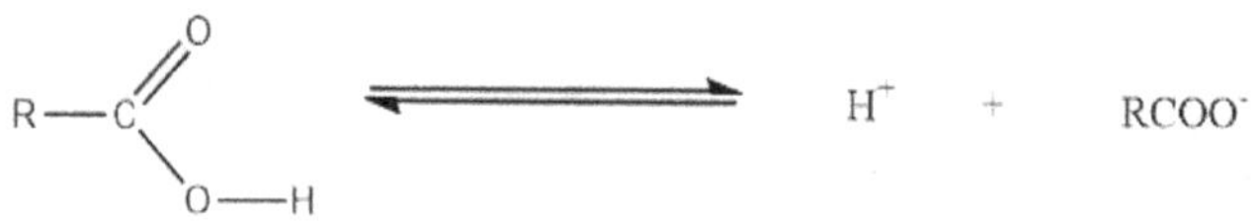

Carboxylic acid   Carboxylate ion

Due to resonance, the carboxylate ion produced following the loss of H^+ ion is stabilised as follows:

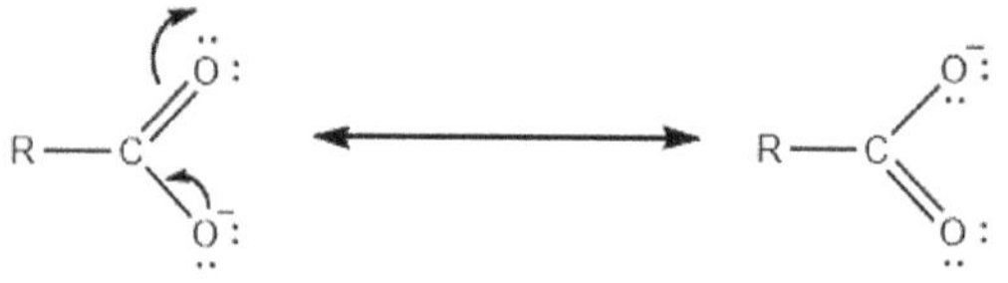

(III)   (IV)

Structures (III) and (IV) are comparable and so contribute equally to the resonance hybrid. As a result, the resonance energy of the carboxylate ion is significantly higher than the resonance energy of the carboxylic acid. In other words, carboxylate ion resonance stabilisation is significantly higher than carboxylic acid resonance stabilisation. Because of its higher stability, the carboxylate ion tends to shift the ionisation process' equilibrium to the right, and therefore is a key contributor in carboxylic acid dissociation. Because the carboxylate ion is a resonance hybrid of equivalent structures (III) and (IV), it may be expressed as follows:

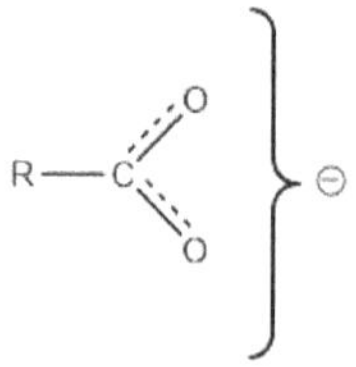

(V)

The above resonance hybrid structure of carboxylate ion is supported by diffraction studies. For instance, in formate ion both the carbon-oxygen bond lengths have the same value (127pm). This is possible because both carbon-oxygen bonds of ion are exactly equivalent.

Molecular orbital theory can also explain the resonating structure. The sp^2 hybridization of the carbonyl carbon is present. These orbitals are in the same plane and point in the same direction as the triangle, forming a 120° angle.

To produce a delocalized π-molecular orbital, the remaining unhybridized p-orbital of the carbon overlaps sidewise with the p-orbitals of both oxygen atoms. In other words, electrons are dispersed about the nuclei of three atoms rather than being confined to the nuclei of two atoms.

This delocalization of π-electrons leads to the stabilization of carboxylate ion and ease of formation of carboxylate ion.

In aqueous solution, carboxylic acids emit H^+ ions, and carboxylic acid is in equilibrium with carboxylate anion and hydronium ion.

$$RCOOH + H_2O \rightleftharpoons RCOO^- + H_3O^-$$

Applying mass of action on the above equation

$$K_c = \frac{[RCOO]^-[H_3O^+]}{[RCOOH][H_2O]}$$

Because water is used in vast quantities and its concentration remains relatively constant, [H2O] may be removed from the preceding equation and the connection recast as:

$$K_a = \frac{[RCOO]^-[H_3O^+]}{[RCOOH]}$$

The equilibrium constant, K_a, is known as acidity constant. K_a tells us about the acidic strength of an acid and therefore it is used as a means for comparing the strengths of different acids.

pK_a values: pK_a value are also used to determine acidic strength of acids. pK_a value is negative logarithm of the acidity constant and is given by:

$$pK_a = -\log K_a$$

A stronger acid has a higher Ka value but a lower pKa value, whereas a weaker acid has a lower Ka but a higher pKa value.

Comparison of acidity of alcohols and carboxylic acids: Both alcohols and carboxylic acids contain -OH group in their molecules but carboxylic acids are strong acids as compared to alcohols. Also, alcohols are practically neutral compounds. This is owing to the carbonyl group (C=O) linked adjacent to the hydroxyl group, which caused the carboxylate ion to gain a negative charge after losing H^+.

The alkoxide ion generated after the loss of H^+ ion in alcohols, on the other hand, is not stabilized due to resonance. As a result, alcohols do not dissociate to a significant degree and are almost rendered virtually neutral.

Comparison of acidity of carboxylic acids and phenols: Carboxylic acids are more powerful than phenolic acids. When the stabilities of carboxylate and phenoxide ions are considered, this can be explained.

In the case of carboxylate ion, the negative charge on the oxygen atom is diffused throughout two oxygen atoms, but the negative charge on the oxygen atom in the case of phenol is only present on one oxygen atom.

Carboxylate ion

Phenoxide ion

The charge delocalization in case of carboxylate ion leads to greater stability and therefore greater ease of formation of carboxylate ion. Therefore, carboxylic acids release H^+ ion easily and are much stronger acids as compared to phenols.

Factors effecting acidity of carboxylic acids

The stability of the products compared to the stability of the reactants determines where the equilibrium is found in the reaction of carboxylic acid and water to produce carboxylate anion and hydronium ion. Variables that stabilise the carboxylate anion more than the carboxylic acid raise the acidity of the carboxylic acid, whereas factors that destabilise the anion lower the acidity.

1. **Electron-releasing alkyl groups**: The acidity of carboxylic acids is reduced by electron-releasing alkyl groups, which enhance the negative charge on the carboxylate ion by releasing electrons and so destabilise it. As a result, the reaction does not go forward, making proton loss harder.

    For example, Acetic acid is weak acid as compared to formic acid.

    Formic Acid

    Acetic Acid

    K_a 17.7×10^{-5} 1.76×10^{-5}

2. **Electron-withdrawing substituents**: Electron-withdrawing substituents like F, Cl, Br, NO2, CN raise the acidity of carboxylic acids by lowering the negative charge on the oxygen atom generated following the removal of H+. This stabilises the carboxylate ion and raises its acidity by making proton removal simpler. Chloroacetic acid, for example, is a much stronger acid than acetic acid.

    Chloroacetic acid

    Acetic Acid

    K_a 136×10^{-5} 1.76×10^{-5}

Fluoroacetic acid is also a stronger acid than chloroacetic acid, according to studies. Furthermore, as the number of electron-withdrawing groups increases, acidity rises.

Chloroacetic acid
K_a 136 x 10^{-5}

Acetic Acid
1.76 x 10^{-5}

Fluoroacetic acid
K_a 260 x 10^{-5}

Chloroacetic acid
136 x 10^{-5}

Trichloroacetic acid
23.200 x 10^{-5}

Dichloroacetic acid
5530 x 10^{-5}

Chloroacetic acid
136 x 10^{-5}

Physical Properties of Carboyxlic Acids

1. Lower carboxylic acids (up to C10) exist as liquids, whereas higher carboxylic acids (up to C10) exist as wax-like solids that are nearly odourless.

2. Carboxylic acids have higher boiling temperatures than alcohols because they create intermolecular hydrogen bonds and hence exist as linked molecules. The boiling point of carboxylic acids rises in lockstep with their molecular weight.

3. Carboxylic acids with an even number of carbon atoms have a greater melting point than homologues with an odd number of carbon atoms, both immediately lower and immediately higher.

   Because carboxyl and terminal methyl groups are on opposing sides of the zig-zag carbon chain in acids with an even number of carbon atoms, this is the case. As a result, they fit together well in the crystal structure, whereas acids with an odd number of carbon atoms have the carboxyl and methyl groups on the same sides of the zig-zag chain, causing them to fit poorly in the crystal structure and having a lower melting temperature.

Even number of carbon atoms
fits better in crystal streuture and hence
have higher melting point

Odd number of carbon atoms
donot fit well in the crystal structure
and hence have lower melting point

4. Due to the creation of intermolecular hydrogen bonds, carboxylic acids exist as dimers.

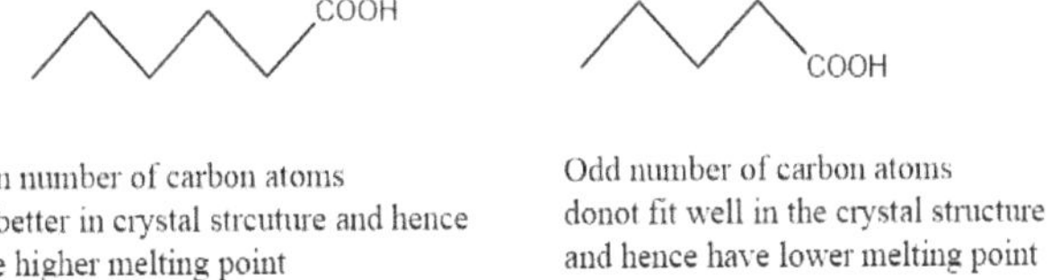

5. Because hydrogen bonds develop with water molecules, lower carboxylic acids are entirely soluble in water. The acid's solubility in water drops significantly as the hydrocarbon chain in the acid lengthens. Organic solvents such as ethanol, ether, and benzene are easily soluble in carboxylic acids.

Methods of Preparation of Carboxylic Acids

1. **Oxidation of primary alcohols or aldehydes:** The oxidation of primary alcohols or aldehydes using oxidising agents such as acidified potassium dichromate, potassium permanganate, or nitric acid produces carboxylic acids.

$$RCH_2OH \text{ or } RCHO \xrightarrow{\;[O]\;} RCOOH$$

Primary alcohol or aldehyde   Carboxylic Acid

Isobutyl alcohol $\xrightarrow{K_2Cr_2O_7,\ H_2SO_4}$ Isobutyric acid

Benzyl alcohol $\xrightarrow{K_2Cr_2O_7,\ H_2SO_4}$ Benzoic Acid

2. **Oxidation of alkylbenzenes:** The alkyl group in alkylbenzenes is oxidised to carbonyl group when heated with oxidising chemicals like acidified potassium dichromate or acidified or alkaline potassium permanganate. Because the alkyl side chain is converted to carboxylic acid regardless of its size, this approach is beneficial for the synthesis of aromatic acids.

Alkyl benzene $\xrightarrow{\;[O]\;}$ Benzoic Acid

Toluene $\xrightarrow[\text{(ii) } H^+]{\text{(i) KMnO}_4/\text{KOH}}$ Benzoic Acid

3. Hydrolysis of nitriles: Carboxylic acids are made by combining nitrile with an aqueous acid or alkali and hydrolyzing it.

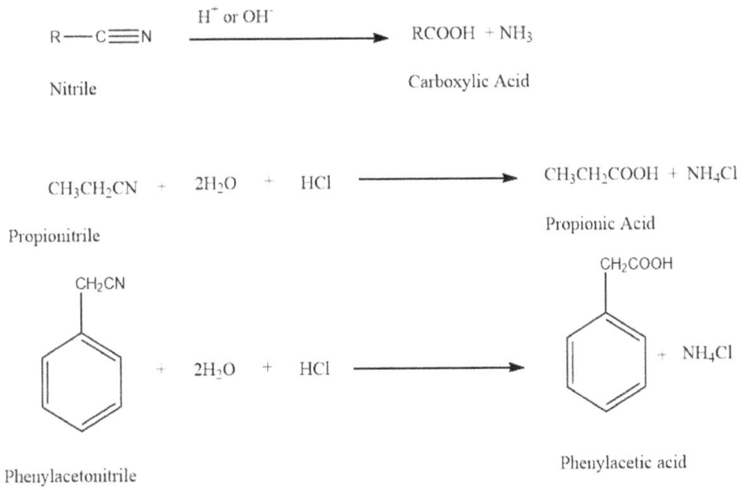

$$R-C\equiv N \xrightarrow{\text{H}^+ \text{ or OH}^-} RCOOH + NH_3$$

Nitrile → Carboxylic Acid

$$CH_3CH_2CN + 2H_2O + HCl \longrightarrow CH_3CH_2COOH + NH_4Cl$$

Propionitrile → Propionic Acid

Phenylacetonitrile + $2H_2O$ + HCl $\longrightarrow$ Phenylacetic acid + NH_4Cl

4. Hydrolysis of acid derivatives such as acid chlorides, anhydrides, esters and amides: Different procedures can be used to convert acid derivatives to carboxylic acid.

Acid chlorides and anhydrides are hydrolyzed in the presence of water, whereas esters and amides are hydrolyzed in the presence of acids or alkalies.

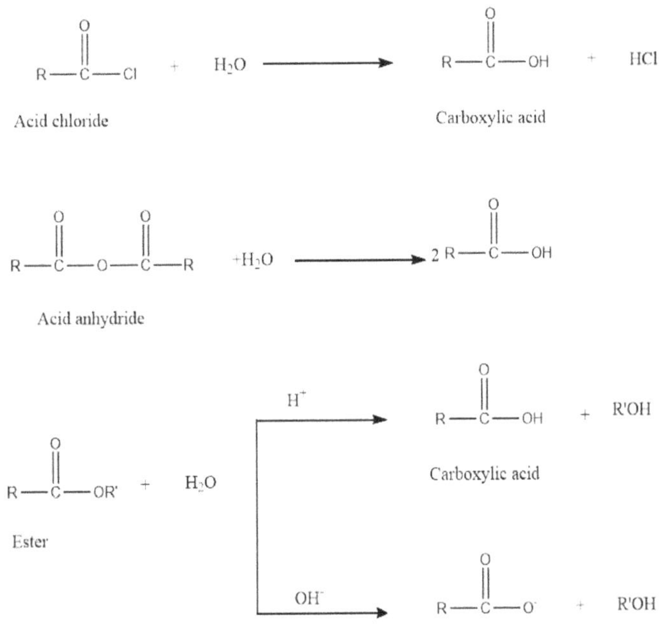

$$\underset{\text{Acid chloride}}{R-\overset{O}{\overset{\|}{C}}-Cl} + H_2O \longrightarrow \underset{\text{Carboxylic acid}}{R-\overset{O}{\overset{\|}{C}}-OH} + HCl$$

$$\underset{\text{Acid anhydride}}{R-\overset{O}{\overset{\|}{C}}-O-\overset{O}{\overset{\|}{C}}-R} + H_2O \longrightarrow 2\ R-\overset{O}{\overset{\|}{C}}-OH$$

$$\underset{\text{Ester}}{R-\overset{O}{\overset{\|}{C}}-OR'} + H_2O \xrightarrow{\text{H}^+} \underset{\text{Carboxylic acid}}{R-\overset{O}{\overset{\|}{C}}-OH} + R'OH$$

$$\xrightarrow{\text{OH}^-} R-\overset{O}{\overset{\|}{C}}-O^- + R'OH$$

5. Carbonation of Grignard reagent: Grignard reagent with carbon dioxide, followed by breakdown of the addition result with dilute acid, can be used to make carboxylic acids. Carbon dioxide can be used in this reaction either as a gas or as solid ice.

$$RMgX + CO_2 \xrightarrow{\text{ether}} RCOOMgX \xrightarrow{H_3O^-} RCOOH$$

Grignard reagent   Addition product   Carboxylic acid

$$H_3C-\underset{\underset{CH_3}{|}}{\overset{\overset{H_2}{\text{C}}}{\text{C}}}-\overset{H}{\text{C}}-MgCl \quad +CO_2 \xrightarrow{\text{Ether}} CH_3\text{-}CH_2\text{-}\underset{\underset{CH_3}{|}}{CH}-COOMgCl$$

Sec-propyl magnesium chloride

$$CH_3\text{-}CH_2\text{-}\underset{\underset{CH_3}{|}}{CH}-COOH + MgCl_2$$

2-methyl butanoic acid

Organolithium compounds can also be used for the preparation of carboxylic acid.

6. **Malonic Ester Synthesis:** A substituted malonic ester is formed by reacting an alkyl halide with the sodium derivative of diethyl malonate. This can be decarboxylated and hydrolyzed to produce an acid.

$$R\text{-}X \quad + \quad Na^-HC\underset{COOC_2H_5}{\overset{COOC_2H_5}{<}} \xrightarrow{-NaX} R-\underset{COOC_2H_5}{\overset{H}{\underset{}{\overset{}{C}}}} \overset{COOC_2H_5}{<}$$

Alkyl halide   Sod. diethyl malonate

$$\xrightarrow{H_2O/H^+}$$

$$RCH_2COOH \xleftarrow[\text{heat}]{-CO_2} R-\underset{COOH}{\overset{H}{C}}\overset{COOH}{<}$$

Carboxylic Acid

7. **Carboxylation of Alkenes**: Heating alkene with carbon monoxide and steam under pressure with phosphoric acid (H_3PO_4) at 400°C produces carboxylic acids. The Koch Reaction is a process for producing carboxylic acids that is widely utilised in industry.

$$CH_2{=}CH_2 \;+\; CO_2 \;+\; H_2O \xrightarrow[\;673K\;]{H_3PO_4} CH_3CH_2COOH$$

Ethene

Propanoic acid

$$CH_3\text{-}CH{=}CH_2 \;+\; CO \;+\; H_2O \xrightarrow[\;673K\;]{H_3PO_4} \underset{\underset{CH_3}{|}}{CH_3\text{-}CH\text{-}COOH}$$

Propene

Isobutyric acid

Qualitative Test of Carboxylic Acids

1. **Ester formation test:** In the presence of strong sulphuric acid, carboxylic acid interacts with alcohol to create ester, which has a fruity odour.

$$R\text{-}COOH \;+\; C_2H_5OH \underset{heat}{\overset{conc.H_2SO_4}{\rightleftharpoons}} R\text{-}COOC_2H_5 \;+\; H_2O$$

Carboxylic acid   Ethanol

Ester

2. **Sodium bicarbonate:** On adding carboxylic acid to saturated solution of sodium bicarbonate, evolution of CO_2 takes place which clearly indicates the presence of carboxylic acid group.

$$R\text{-}COOH \;+\; NaHCO_3 \longrightarrow RCOONa \;+\; H_2O \;+\; CO_2$$

Carboxylic Acid

Sodium salt

Chemical Reactions of Carboxylic Acids

Carboxyl group has both carbonyl and hydroxyl groups, therefore it should exhibit qualities of both functional groups. However, it has been discovered that carbonyl group does not react with nucleophilic chemicals. The carbonyl group, on the other hand, has an effect on the behaviour of the hydroxyl group and is responsible for the acidic nature of the hydroxyl group's hydrogen.

1. **Acidity:** Carboxylic acids are acidic in nature, releasing H+ ions in aqueous solution and coexisting with the carboxylate anion and the hydronium ion in equilibrium.

$$RCOOH \;+\; H_2O \rightleftharpoons RCOO^- \;+\; H_3O^-$$

Carboxylic acid

Carboxylate ion

2. **Salt formation:** Carboxylic acids form salts and liberate hydrogen when they react with strongly electropositive metals like sodium, potassium, and zinc.

$$2RCOOH \;+\; 2Na \longrightarrow 2RCOONa \;+\; H_2$$

Carboxylic acid

Sodium carboxylate

$$2CH_3COOH \;+\; Zn \longrightarrow (CH_3COO)_2Zn \;+\; H_2$$

Acetic acid

Zinc acetate

3. **Formation of esters**: Carboxylic acids create esters when they are treated with alcohols in the presence of a strong mineral (such as HCl or H_2SO_4) or a Lewis acid (such as BF_3). The reaction is known as esterification because it is reversible in nature.

$$RCOOH + R'OH \underset{H^+}{\rightleftharpoons} RCOOR' + H_2O$$

Carboxylic acid   Alcohol   Ester

$$CH_3COOH + C_2H_5OH \underset{H^+}{\rightleftharpoons} CH_3COOC_2H_5 + H_2O$$

Acetic acid   Ethyl alcohol   Ethyl acetate

The process of esterification is very difficult to carry out if the acid or alcohol used in the reaction contains bulky group near the -COOH or -OH group because steric hindrance is caused by such bulky groups hence it is very difficult to bring about an esterification reaction involving a tertiary alcohol.

As a result, in the esterification reaction, the order of reactivity of alcohols is:

Primary> secondary > tertiary

4. **Formation of acid chlorides**: The hydroxyl group of carboxylic acids is replaced by chlorine when they are treated with phosphorus pentachloride, phosphorus trichloride, or thionyl chloride, resulting in acid chlorides.

$$RCOOH + PCl_5 \longrightarrow RCOCl + POCl_3 + HCl$$

$$3RCOOH + PCl_3 \longrightarrow 3RCOCl + H_3PO_3$$

$$RCOOH + SOCl_2 \longrightarrow RCOCl + SO_2 + HCl$$

5. **Formation of amides:** When carboxylic acids are treated with ammonia, they generate ammonium salts, which lose a molecule of water when heated to generate amides.

$$RCOOH + NH_3 \longrightarrow RCOONH_4 \xrightarrow[-H_2O]{Heat} RCONH_2$$

Ammonium salt   Acid amide

6. **Formation of anhydrides**: The formation of matching anhydrides when carboxylic acids are treated with acid chlorides in the presence of pyridine.

$$RCOOH + RCOCl + Pyridine \longrightarrow$$

Carboxylic acid   Acid chloride

acid anhydride

+ Pyridine hydrochloride

$$CH_3COOH + CH_3COCl + Pyridine \longrightarrow$$

Acetic acid   Acetyl chloride

Acetic anhydride

+ Pyridine hydrochloride

7. **Reduction**: Carboxylic acids can be reduced by lithium aluminium hydride to form primary alcohols. During reduction carboxyl group is reduced to CH_2.

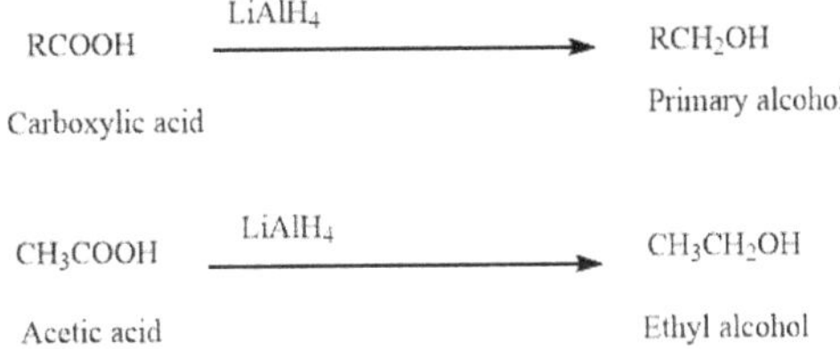

8. **Decarboxylation:** When sodium salts of carboxylic acids are heated with sodalime (NaOH + CaO), the carboxylic acids are decarboxylated and hydrocarbons are formed.

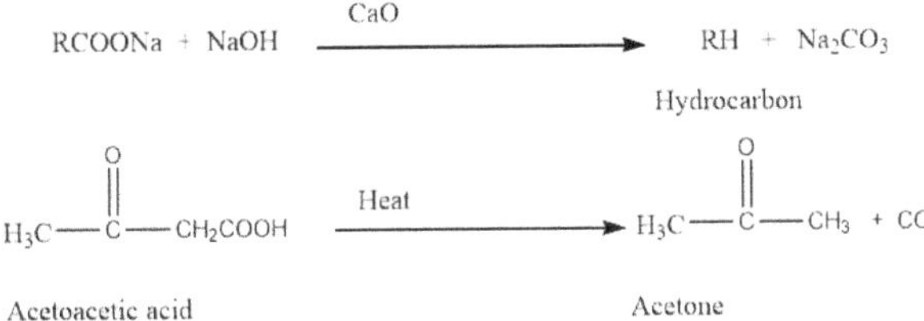

It may be noted that carboxylic acids containing electron-withdrawing groups such as $-NO_2$ and CH_3CO^- get decarboxylated just by heating alone.

9. **(i) Kolbe's electrolytic reaction**: Alkali salts of carboxylic acids on electrolysis get decarboxylated to form hydrocarbons.

   1. Alkanes are obtained by electrolysis of a concentrated aqueous solution of sodium or potassium salts of monocarboxylic acids.

$$2RCOONa + 2H_2O \xrightarrow{\text{Electrolysis}} R-R + 2NaOH + H_2$$
$$\text{Alkane}$$

The reaction takes place as follows:

$$2RCOONa \rightleftharpoons 2RCOO^- + 2Na^-$$
Sodium salt of acid

$$2H_2O \rightleftharpoons 2H^- + 2OH^-$$

At the anode
$$2RCOO^- \longrightarrow 2RCOO+2e^- \longrightarrow R\text{-}R + 2CO_2$$
$$\text{Alkane}$$

At the cathode
$$2H+ 2e- \longrightarrow H_2$$

When compared to Na+ ions, H+ ions have a lower discharge potential. As a result, H+ ions are released at the cathode, releasing H_2, while Na+ ions stay in solution.

This is a good way to make ethane and other higher alkanes with an even number of carbon atoms.

Methane cannot be prepared by this method.

(ii) Decarboxylation of monocarboxylic acid- Sodium salts of monocarboxylic acids undergo decarboxylation when heated with soda lime (NaOH+ CaO) with liberation of carbon dioxide from carboxylic group.

$$RCOONa + NaOH \xrightarrow{CaO} RH + Na_2CO_3$$

Sodium salt of acid   Alkane

$$CH_3COONa + NaOH \longrightarrow CH_4 + Na_2CO_3$$

Sodium acetate   Methane

10. **Decarboxylative halogenation (Hunsdiecker reaction):** In a carbon tetrachloride solution, a silver salt of carboxylic acid is decomposed by chlorine or bromine to generate an alkyl or aryl halide with one carbon atom less than the original acid.

$$RCOOAg + Br_2 \xrightarrow[\text{reflux, 350K}]{CCl_4} R\text{-}Br + AgBr + CO_2$$

Silver salt of
carboxylic acid

$$CH_3COOAg + Br_2 \xrightarrow[\text{reflux, 350K}]{CCl_4} CH_3Br + AgBr + CO_2$$

Silver acetate   Bromomethane

11. **Halogenation of alkyl groups:** The -hydrogen atoms of alkyl groups of aliphatic acids are replaced by chlorine or bromine when carboxylic acids with -hydrogen are treated with bromine in the presence of modest amounts of red phosphorus to generate a haloacid. The Hell-Volhard Zelinsky reaction, or HVZ reaction, is the name given to this reaction.

$$CH_3CH_2COOH \xrightarrow[-HBr]{Br_2/P} CH_3CHBrCOOH \xrightarrow[-HBr]{Br_2/P} CH_3CBr_2COOH$$

Propanoic acid   α–Bromopropanoic acid   α,α–Dibromopropanoic acid

Qualitative Test of Amides

1. **Sodium hydroxide test:** When small amount of amide is treated with few drops of sodium hydroxide and then boiled, there is evolution of ammonia gas which turns red litmus to blue.

$$RCONH_2 + NaOH \longrightarrow RCOONa + NH_3$$

Amide   Sodium salt of carboxylic   Ammonia
                                      acid

2. **Hydroxamic acid test:** A bluish red colour is formed when a small sample of amide is treated with hydroxylamine and heated over a water bath for five minutes before cooling and adding a few drops of alcoholic ferric chloride, confirming the presence of an amide group.

3. **Nitrous acid test**: In small sample of amide, few drops of dil. HCl are added followed by addition of sodium nitrite solution, brisk effervescene due to evolution of nitrogen gas which confirms the presence of amide group.

$$RCONH_2 + NH_2OH.HCl \longrightarrow R-\overset{O}{\underset{}{C}}-\overset{H}{\underset{}{N}}-OH + NH_3$$

Amide — ammonium hydroxide hydrochloride — Hydroxamic acid

$$R-\overset{O}{\underset{}{C}}-\overset{H}{\underset{}{N}}-OH + FeCl_3 \longrightarrow \left(R-\overset{O}{\underset{}{C}}-NHO\right)_3 Fe + 3HCl$$

Hydroxamic acid — Bluish red colour

$$NaNO_2(s) + HCl(aq) \longrightarrow NaCl + O=N-OH$$

Nitrous Acid

$$R-\overset{O}{\underset{}{C}}-NH_2 + HNO_2 \longrightarrow RCOOH + H_2O + N_2 \text{ (evolves)}$$

Amide — Nitrous Acid

Qualitative Test of Esters

1. **Phenolphthalein test:** When small sample of ester is dissolved in water with few drops of phenolphthalein with addition of few drops of dil. NaOH solution followed by heating till the disappearance of pink colour indicates the presence of ester.

$$RCOOR' \underset{}{\overset{OH^-}{\rightleftharpoons}} RCOOH + R'OH$$

Ester — carboxylic acid   alcohol

Carboxylic acid produced lowers down the pH of the solution and hence colour of solution changes from pink to colourless

2. **Hydroxamic test:** When small sample of ester is treated with hydroxylamine in ethanol followed by addition of sodium hydroxide and heating with addition of HCl and $FeCl_3$, deep red colour is obtained which shows the presence of ester.

$$R-\overset{O}{\underset{}{C}}-OR' + NH_2OH \overset{OH^-}{\longrightarrow} R-\overset{O}{\underset{}{C}}-\overset{H}{\underset{}{N}}-OH$$

$$\downarrow FeCl_3$$

$$\left(R-\underset{O}{\overset{}{C}}-NHO\right)_3 + 3HCl$$

Reddish blue colour

Structure and uses of Carboxylic Acids

Acetic acid

Chemical formula: CH₃COOH

$$H_3C-\overset{\overset{\displaystyle O}{\|}}{C}-OH$$

1. Acetic acid is an antibiotic that is used to treat bacterial and fungal infections.
2. Infections in the ear canal are treated with acetic acid (for the ear).
3. In many parts of the developing world, acetic acid can be administered to the cervix to aid in the detection of cervical cancer during screening.
4. In various manufacturing processes for the creation of substrates, acetic acid is employed as a chemical reagent for the creation of a variety of chemical compounds such as acetic anhydride, ester, vinyl acetate monomer, vinegar, and many more polymeric products. It's commonly used to purify organic molecules and can also be used to recrystallize them.
5. Acetic acid is used in a variety of medical applications. Its most prominent application is as an antiseptic against pseudomonas, enterococci, streptococci, staphylococci, and other bacteria. It's also employed in breast cancer screening and illness prevention. Red blood cells, on the other hand, are utilised to lyse white blood cells before they are examined. It's also been claimed that vinegar helps to lower blood sugar levels.
6. Vinegar is often made from acetic acid, a diluted solvent. As we all know, vinegar is often used for washing, laundry, cooking, and a variety of other household tasks. Farmers have traditionally sprayed acetic acid on animal silage to prevent bacterial and fungal growth. Acetic acid is also employed in the production of inks and dyes, as well as the production of perfumes. It's also in the rubber and plastics processing industries.

Lactic acid: CH₃CH(OH)COOH

$$H_3C-\overset{\overset{\displaystyle OH}{|}}{\underset{\underset{\displaystyle H}{|}}{C}}-\overset{\overset{\displaystyle O}{\|}}{C}-OH$$

1. Lactic acid is an emollient that can be used to treat dry, scaly skin disorders like xerosis and ichthyosis vulgaris, as well as reduce itching.
2. Lactic acid is used to treat hyperpigmentation, age spots, and other conditions that cause a dull, uneven complexion. Improved skin tone and pore appearance are two further advantages of AHAs like lactic acid.
3. It is utilised in the food and pharmaceutical industries.
4. It is utilised in the manufacture of polymers.
5. It aids in the coagulation of milk protein.
6. It is used in the colouring of textiles and the tanning of leather.
7. Lactate is essential for the recovery of traumatic brain lesions.
8. Lactate triggers the release of norepinephrine in the brain.

Tartaric acid:

Structure: COOHCH(OH)CH(OH)COOH or$C_4H_6O_6$

$$
\begin{array}{c}
OH \\
|\\
HC-COOH \\
|\\
HC-COOH \\
|\\
OH
\end{array}
$$

1. Because of its antioxidant characteristics, tartaric acid is easily soluble in water and widely employed in the food sector.
2. Tartaric acid has a variety of industrial uses, including metal polishing, photographic printing, and wool dyeing.
3. Tartaric acid is commonly found in carbonated beverages, effervescent pills, gelatin desserts, and fruit jellies as an acidulant.
4. Cream of tartar is used in the cleaning of brass, the electrolytic tinning of iron and steel, and the coating of other metals with gold and silver. It is also used in baking powders, hard candies, and taffies.
5. Tartar emetic is employed as a pesticide as well as a mordant for dyeing.
6. Tartaric acid is one of the least antibacterial organic acids, with fewer bacteria inactivated and microbial development inhibited.

Citric acid:

Molecular formula: $C_6H_8O_7$

$$
\begin{array}{c}
COOH \\
|\\
CH_2 \\
|\\
HOOC-C-OH \\
|\\
CH_2 \\
|\\
COOH
\end{array}
$$

Uses:

1. Citric acid is used to reduce the acidity of urine. Less acidic urine aids in the removal of uric acid from the kidneys, reducing the risk of gout and some types of kidney stones (urate). This medicine can also be used to prevent and treat some metabolic disorders caused by renal disease (acidosis).
2. Citric acid is frequently used in the manufacture of packaged foods and beverages. It aids in the preservation of canned and jarred goods over extended periods of time. It can help keep some fresh-cut vegetables from browning, such as sliced apples. Citric acid can also thicken meals or impart a somewhat sour flavour to them. That's why some ice creams, sorbets, and sodas have citric acid listed as an ingredient.
3. Alcoholic beverages. Citric acid can counteract the acidity of a meal or beverage. Winemakers use it to enhance the flavour of their products.

4. Pharmaceuticals. Citric acid is found in several lotions to aid in the healing of skin infections. Other oral citric acid medications can help to reduce the quantity of acid in your urine. This may aid in the prevention of kidney stones. Citric acid can also be used to treat metabolic acidosis, which is a buildup of acid in the body.

5. Dietary supplements Calcium citrate pills, which can help avoid kidney stones, are taken by some persons.

6. Personal-care items. When citric acid is combined with other chemicals, a "alpha hydroxy acid" molecule is formed, which helps to smooth your skin. It's included in several cosmetics and toiletries to help them last longer, such as lipstick, hair spray, and deodorant.

7. Cleaners for the home. Citric acid is commonly found in dishwasher detergent because it can break down hard water buildup. It's also an ingredient in other household cleansers because it may help eliminate stains and odours.

8. Disinfectants are number eight on the list. Citric acid is used in insect sprays, fungus or algae-killing treatments, hand sanitizer, and even some tissues used to blow your nose because it destroys some bacteria and viruses.

9. Cleaning goods for the environment. Citric acid has the ability to safely remove pollutants from polluted soil as well as clean up nuclear waste.

Succinic acid

Molecular formula: $C_4H_6O_4$

$$CH_2COOH$$
$$|$$
$$CH_2COOH$$

Uses:

1. Succinic acid is a component of some alkyd resins and a precursor to several polyesters. [10] Succinic acid can be used as a precursor to make 1,4-butanediol (BDO).

2. BDO is a major supplier of connectors, insulators, wheel covers, gearshift knobs, and reinforcing beams to the automotive and electronics sectors.

3. Succinic acid is also used as a base in the production of biodegradable polymers that are useful in tissue engineering.

4. Succinic acid is largely employed in the food and beverage industries as an acidity regulator[20]. It can also be used as a flavouring agent, adding a sour and astringent element to the umami flavour.

5. It's utilised as an excipient in pharmaceuticals to regulate acidity[21] and as a counter ion.

Oxalic acid

Molecular formula:$C_2H_2O_4$

$$COOH$$
$$|$$
$$COOH$$
$.2H_2O$

Uses:

1. As previously stated, oxalic acid is mostly utilised for the most difficult cleaning tasks. The acid has bleach-like properties and can be used to remove rust and stains from metals and

objects. Several cleaning solutions, detergents, and bleaches include this acid in some form. Oxalic acid can also be used to polish almost any stone and to treat aged wood.

2. This chemical is mostly used in industry for mineral processing procedures. Oxalic acid can also be used to disinfect equipment, and those working in the textile industry use it to bleach clothes.

3. In the medical field, corporations use the acid to further purify or dilute particular compounds. However, there is a scarcity of information about this acid's health benefits. Oxalic acid is non-lethal in both organic and raw forms. However, it can sometimes have negative consequences in the body.

4. Oxalic acid is mostly utilised as a reducing element in developing photographic film, in addition to bleaching, eliminating rust, and staining. This acid is also utilised in wastewater treatment, where it successfully dissolves calcium deposits from water.

5. In lanthanide chemistry, oxalic acid is an important reagent. In very strongly acidic solutions, hydrated lanthanide oxalates form rapidly in a densely crystalline, easily filtered form that is mainly free of nonlanthanide elements. The oxides, which are the most generally marketed form of these elements, are formed by the thermal decomposition of this oxalate.

6. Cleaning and bleaching are two of oxalic acid's most common uses, particularly for rust removal (iron complexing agent). Because it forms a stable, water-soluble salt with ferric iron, ferrioxalate ion, it is useful in rust removal agents.

Salicylic acid

Molecular formula: $C_7H_6O_3$

1. Salicylic acid is a medicine that aids in the removal of the skin's outer layer. Warts, calluses, psoriasis, dandruff, acne, ringworm, and ichthyosis are all treated with it.

2. Some "skin-reddening" products contain salicylic acid and its derivatives.

3. Salicylic acid has keratolytic properties (peeling agent). Salicylic acid causes the outer layer of skin to slough.

4. Salicylic acid topical (skin) is used to treat acne, dandruff, seborrhea, and psoriasis, as well as corns, calluses, and warts.

5. A beta hydroxy acid is salicylic acid. It's well-known for eliminating acne and keeping pores clear by exfoliating the skin. Salicylic acid is found in a number of over-the-counter (OTC) medications. Prescription-strength formulations are also available.

6. Salicylic acid is the best treatment for mild acne (blackheads and whiteheads). It may also aid in the prevention of subsequent outbreaks.

Benzoic acid

Molecular formula: C_6H_5COOH

Uses:

1. Benzoic acid is a chemical that is utilised in medicine. It's utilised in pharmaceuticals as a preservative. It's also in baby products, skin care products, cleansing products, hair and nail care products, soaps, bath products, and detergents, among other things.

2. It helps to keep bacterial infections at bay. It's an antifungal that's used to treat infections like ringworm and athlete's foot. After conjugation with glycine in the liver, it is eliminated as hippuric acid. Hippuric acid discharged is not poisonous. It is used to relieve skin irritation caused by bug bites, burns, and other factors.

3. Foods that contain naturally occurring benzoic acid, such as ripe cloves, berries, and cinnamon. Food preservation involves the use of benzoic acid. Salad dressings, soft drinks, fruit juices, and pickles are just a few examples. Benzoic acid is commonly found in processed foods to inhibit the growth of bacteria, mould, and yeast.

4. Benzoic acid is most typically encountered in industrial settings, where it is used to make perfumes, dyes, topical treatments, and insect repellents, among other things.

5. Benzoate plasticizers such glycol, diethylene glycol, and triethylene glycol esters are made by transesterifying methyl benzoate with the appropriate diol. These compounds can also be produced by reacting benzoyl chloride with a diol. These plasticizers are used in the same way that terephthalic acid ester plasticizers are.

6. Whitfield's ointment contains benzoic acid, which is used to treat fungal skin infections such as tinea, ringworm, and athlete's foot. Benzoic acid is a prominent component of both tincture of benzoin and Friar's balsam, as it is the main component of gum benzoin. Topical antiseptics and inhalant decongestants have long been used with these goods.

Benzyl Benzoate

Molecular formula: $C_{14}H_{12}O_2$

Uses:

1. Benzyl benzoate is a topical therapy for human scabies that is both effective and affordable.

2. It is found in many asthma and whooping cough medications and has vasodilating and spasmolytic properties.

3. It's also an excipient in several testosterone-replacement drugs (like Nebido) for hypogonadism treatment.

4. In veterinary hospitals, benzyl benzoate is used as a topical acaricide, scabicide, and pediculicide.

5. Benzyl benzoate is utilised as a chigger, tick, and mosquito repellent. In the perfume industry, it's also utilised as a dye carrier, cellulose derivatives solvent, plasticizer, and fixative.

6. Benzyl benzoate is used to treat infestations of lice and scabies. This medication is said to be absorbed by lice and mites, killing them by working on their nerve systems.

Dimethyl phthalate

Chemical formula: $(C_2H_3O_2)_2C_6H_4$

Uses:

1. Mosquitoes and flies are repellents made from dimethyl phthalate. It's also an ectoparasiticide with a variety of different applications, such as solid rocket propellants and polymers.

2. Used in the production of polymers, insect repellents, safety glass, and lacquer coatings, among other things.

3. In humans and animals, acute (short-term) inhalation exposure to dimethyl phthalate causes irritation of the eyes, nose, and throat.

4. This synthetic chemical is often used to increase the flexibility of plastics. It can be found in toothbrushes, vehicle parts, tools, toys, and food packaging, among other things. Because it is not part of the chemical chain (polymers) that makes up the plastic, diethyl phthalate can be easily removed from these items. Cosmetics, pesticides, and aspirin all contain diethyl phthalate.

5. Solid rocket propellants, lacquers, plastics, safety glasses, rubber coating agents, moulding powders, insect repellants, and pesticides all include dimethyl phthalate.

6. It's employed in cellulose acetate, polyvinyl fluoride coating repellant agents, and solvents as a plasticizer.

7. Dimethyl Phthalate is a solvent as well as a rodenticide rat poison, rat completed, chlorine mouse ketone intermediates.

8. The product is a plasticizer for a wide range of resins with a high dissolving power that is compatible with cellulose resin, rubber, and vinyl resin. It has good film-forming, adhesion, and water resistance properties. In the creation of cellulose acetate film, varnish, translucent paper, and moulding powder, it is commonly combined with diethyl phthalate. Nitrocellulose is made with a tiny amount of the product. The product can also be used as a nitrile rubber

plasticizer, and it has strong cold resistance. Other plasticizers might be added in with the product. It has the ability to overcome excessive volatility, low-temperature crystallisation, and other flaws. DEET oil (crude oil) and DDT solvents are also made from the goods. The product is also utilised as a stationary phase in gas chromatography.

Methyl salicylate

Molecular formula: $C_8H_8O_3$

Uses:

1. In deep heating liniments, methyl salicylate is utilised as a rubefacient and analgesic.
2. It is used as an antibacterial in mouthwash solutions and as a flavouring additive in chewing gums and mints in tiny doses.
3. It's utilised in mouthwash as an antiseptic.
4. It is used to provide aroma to a variety of products and to hide the odour of some organophosphate pesticides.
5. Methyl salicylate is also utilised as a bait to attract male orchid bees for research, as the molecule is thought to be used to make pheromones.
6. Methyl salicylate is utilised as a rubefacient and analgesic in deep heating liniments for acute joint and muscular pain. It's used in small amounts as a flavouring agent in chewing gums and mints, and as an antibacterial in mouthwash solutions.

Acetyl salicylic acid

Molecular formula: $C_9H_8O_4$

Uses:

1. Aspirin is used to treat a variety of ailments, including fever, pain, rheumatic fever, and inflammatory illnesses such rheumatoid arthritis, pericarditis, and Kawasaki disease. Lower aspirin doses have also been found to reduce the risk of death from a heart attack or stroke in persons who are at high risk or have cardiovascular disease, but not in otherwise healthy older individuals. Although the mechanisms of aspirin's anti-cancer impact are unknown, there is some evidence that it can help prevent colorectal cancer.
2. Aspirin's ability to regulate fever is owing to its irreversible suppression of COX in the prostaglandin pathway.

3. Aspirin is an anti-inflammatory drug used to treat both acute and chronic inflammation, as well as inflammatory illnesses like rheumatoid arthritis.
4. Aspirin is thought to lower the overall risk of cancer, as well as the likelihood of dying from it. This impact is especially favourable in the case of colorectal cancer (CRC).
5. Aspirin is the first-line treatment for acute rheumatic fever's fever and joint pain.
6. In veterinary medicine, aspirin is sometimes used as an anticoagulant or to treat pain caused by musculoskeletal inflammation or osteoarthritis. Because adverse effects, such as gastro-intestinal problems, are widespread, aspirin should only be given to animals under the direct supervision of a veterinarian.

Amines:

Amines are ammonia derivatives that have one or more hydrogens replaced with alkyl or aryl groups.

For example,

Methylamine	Dimethylamine	Trimethylamine

Classification of amines:

Primary, secondary, and tertiary amines are distinguished by the replacement of one, two, or three hydrogen atoms in ammonia.

(a) **Primary amines**: Primary amines are those in which an alkyl or aryl group replaces one hydrogen of ammonia, R. The presence of an amino group, -NH2, linked to an alkyl or aryl group, R, is used to identify primary groups.

CH_3NH_2

Methylamine

Aryl amine

(b) **Secondary amines**: Secondary amines are those that have two alkyl or aryl groups in place of two hydrogens in ammonia. An iminogroup, -NH-, is connected to two alkyl or aryl groups in secondary amines. The amine is called simple if the two alkyl or aryl groups attached are same, whereas the amine is called mixed amine if the alkyl or aryl groups are different.

Dimethylamine

N-methylaniline

Diphenylamine

(c) Tertiary amines: All three hydrogens of ammonia have been replaced by alkyl or aryl groups in tertiary amines. The N atom is connected to three alkyl or aryl groups in tertiary amines.

Trimethylamine   N.N-dimethylaniline

Structure of amines:

Amines have a similar structure to ammonia. The sp3hybridized orbitals of the nitrogen atom in ammonia are pointed towards the tetrahedron's corners. Three of these orbitals have a single electron, forming a sigma bond with the alkyl or aryl group. A lone pair of electrons can be found in the fourth sp3hybridised orbital. Amines have a pyramidal form with a bond angle of 109.5°, but trimethylamine has a bond angle of 108° due to stronger steric repulsion between methyl groups than between hydrogen atoms in ammonia.

Physical properties of amines:

1. **Physical state**: Lower alipthatic amines are gases with an ammonia-like odour, while higher alipthatic amines are mainly liquids with fishy odours. Pure amines are colourless, but they discolour when exposed to oxygen.

2. **Melting and boiling points**: Because amines may form intermolecular hydrogen bonds, they have higher boiling temperatures than non-polar molecules of comparable molecular weight. However, intermolecular hydrogen bonding in amines is weaker than intermolecular hydrogen bonding in alcohols, thus we may conclude that amines have a greater boiling point than non-polar compounds but a lower boiling point than alcohols.

3. Amines are water soluble due to their ability to create hydrogen bonds with water. The higher amines, on the other hand, are water insoluble due to the increase in the size of the non-polar hydrocarbon component.

Intermolecular hydrogen bonding

Separation of Primary, Secondary and Tertiary amines

Various ways for separating a combination of primary amines, secondary amines, and tertiary amines are given below:

(i) **Fractional distillation**: Because their boiling points differ, fractional distillation can be used to separate mixtures of primary, secondary, and tertiary amines using extremely efficient fractionating apparatus.

(ii) **Hofmann's method**: When a mixture of amines is exposed to diethyl oxalate, primary amines create a substituted oxamide (a solid), secondary amines form dialkyloxamic ester (a liquid), and tertiary amines have no reaction.

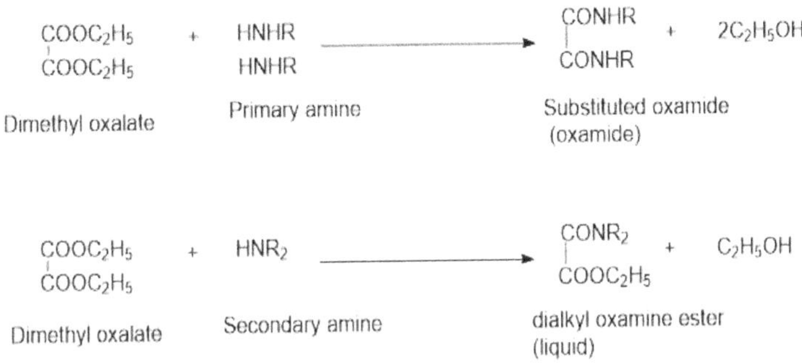

Regeneration of amines: The reaction mixture is now fractionally distilled, tertiary amines distills first followed by dialkyloxamine ester and finally oxamide remains behind the distillation flask.

The oxamine and oxamide are further hydrolysed with KOH to give back the amines which are distilled off.

(iii) **Hinsberg's method**: In the presence of sodium hydroxide, the amine mixture is treated with p-toluenesulphonyl chloride, also known as tosyl chloride (TSCl) or Hinsberg's reagent.

The **primary amines** react with mono-alkyl sulphonamide which dissolves in sodium hydroxide with the formation of sodium salt.

CH₃

+ H₂NR $\xrightarrow[-HCl]{}$

p-Toulene sulphonyl chloride

CH₃

SO₂NHR
N-alkyl sulphonamide

NaOH

CH₃

+ H₂O

SO₂NR
Na

Sod. salt of N-alkyl sulphonamide (Soluble)

Diakylsulphonamide is formed by secondary amines and is insoluble in alkali.

CH₃

SO₂Cl

+ NHR₂ $\longrightarrow$

p-Toulene sulphonyl chloride

CH₃

SO₂NR₂

+ HCl

N,N-dialkyl sulphonamide
(Insoluble in alkali)

The tertiary amines have no reaction.

On the basis of product obtained it is possible to distinguish between various classes of amines.

Basicity of amines:

Amines are basic in nature due to the presence of a lone pair of electrons on the nitrogen atom, which is available for donation to Lewis acids such as BH3, AlCl3, and others, as well as protonation.

$$RNH_2 \; + \; H_2O \; \rightleftharpoons \; RNH_3^+ \; + \; OH^-$$

Basicity constants: Strong bases are those that totally ionise in aqueous solution, such as sodium hydroxide and potassium hydroxide. Amines, on the other hand, are weaker bases that only partially ionise in aqueous solutions, resulting in a state of equilibrium between the ionised and un-ionized forms.

The convenient way of expressing the basicity of amines is in terms of equilibrium constants, K_b called basicity constant which is derived from above equation as:

$$K_b = \frac{[RNH_3^+][OH^-]}{RNH_2}$$

In above equation concentration of water has been ignored because it remains practically constant.

The basicity constant is a measure of a weak base's relative strength. Basicity constants have greater numerical values for stronger bases, while they have lower numerical values for weaker bases.

Ammonia is less basic than aliphatic amines because the alkyl group linked to the nitrogen atom has a +I effect, which raises the electron density on nitrogen and makes electrons more readily available for donation, lowering its basicity.

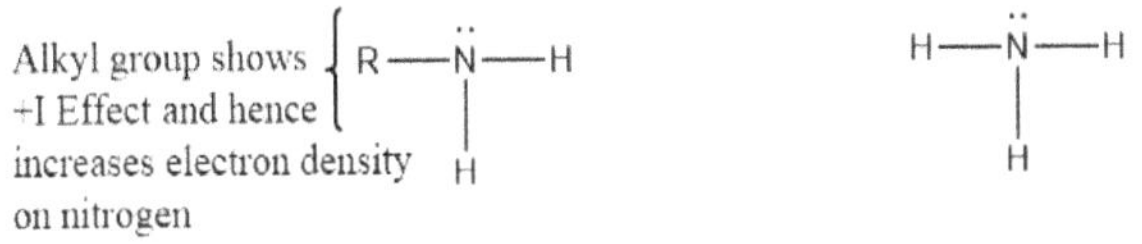

Aliphatic amines

Ammonia

Relative basicity of amines: The availability of lone pair electrons on nitrogen atom determines amine basicity, and factors that enhance the availability of electron pair on nitrogen or improve the stability of ammonium ion relative to parent amine would enhance amine basicity. Any condition that reduces the availability of electron pairs on nitrogen or the stability of the ammonium ion relative to the parent amine, on the other hand, reduces the basicity of amines. The following are some of the factors that influence amine basicity:

(i) **Inductive effect**: Aliphatic amines have one or more alkyl groups connected to them in place of ammonia hydrogen atoms. Alkyl groups now have a +I impact because they release electrons in nature, making the electron pair on the nitrogen atom more available for sharing.

Also, the electron releasing effect of alkyl groups decreases the positive charge of the substituted ammonium ion formed by amine and thus increases its stability.

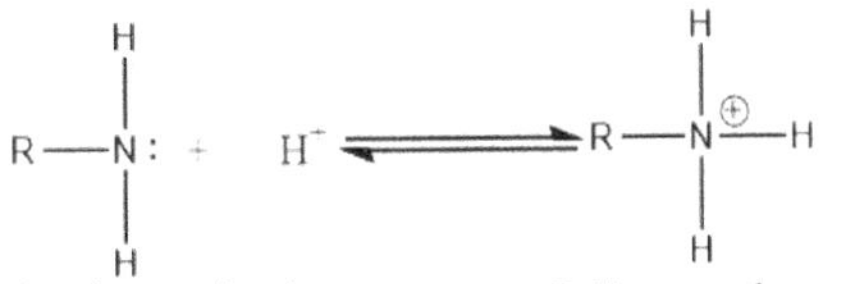

Alkyl groups increases the electron density around nitrogen and hence increases its basicity

R disperses the positive charge of ammonium ion and hence stabilizes it

Hence it is expected that tertiary amines should be strongest base followed by secondary amines and primary amines whereas experimentally it has been found that tertiary amines are weaker bases as compared to secondary amines as well as primary amines.

Relative order of basicity of amines according to Inductive effect:

$$(CH_3)_3N > (CH_3)_2NH > (CH_3)NH_2$$

Actual order of basicity of amines found experimentally:

$$(CH_3)_2NH > (CH_3)NH_2 > (CH_3)_3N.$$

This clearly indicates that relative basicity of amines cannot be described solely by the inductive effect, and that additional aspects such as solvation effects must also be considered.

(ii) Solvation effect: The aliphatic amines' relative stability is explained in part by the solubility effect. The ammonium ion generated following aliphatic amine protonation is stabilised by solvation in water via hydrogen bonding. The number of hydrogen atoms in substituted amines that may establish hydrogen bonds determines the extent of solvation and subsequent stabilisation, as shown:

ammonium ion formed 1^0 amine gets stabilised maximum through solvation

ammonium ion formed from 2^0 amines

Ammonum ion formed from 3^0 amine, minimum stablised through solvation

As the number of hydrogen atoms on substituted ammonium ion decreasing on going from 1° to 3° amine, the extent of stabilization of the ion by solvation also decreases.

Thus, basicity order of amines on basis of solvation effect alone should be:

$$(CH_3)NH_2 > (CH_3)_2NH > (CH_3)_3N.$$

Therefore, solvation effect and inductive effect has opposing influence on the basicity of amines.

Because solvation is lowest and steric hinderance is highest in 3° amine, it is least basic despite having the greatest inductive impact.

The steric hinderance is lowest in 1° amine, the solvation effect is highest, and the inductive effect is lowest. As a result, its basic strength exceeds 3° amine.

All of these factors combine to make 2° amine more basic than 1° amine.

As a result, general basic strength ranges from 2° > 1° > 3°.

Qualitative test for amines:

Below given methods can be used for the Qualitative estimation of amines.

1. Carbylamine test: When primary amine interacts with chloroform and alcoholic potash, it forms an alkyl isocyanide (or carbylamine), which has a strong odour.

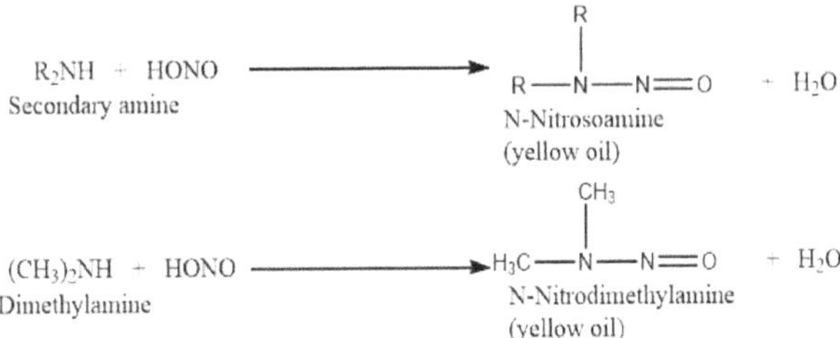

$$R\text{-}NH_2 \ + \ CHCl_3 + \ 3KOH \longrightarrow R\text{---}\overset{+}{N}\overset{-}{\equiv}C \ + \ 3KCl \ + \ 3H_2O$$

1^0 amine   Isocyanate

This reaction can be used for the qualitative estimation of amines.

2. **Reaction with nitrous acid**: The three classes of amines react with nitrous acid to produce three distinct compounds, as follows:

(a) Diaznoum salts are formed when primary aliphatic amines combine with cold nitrous acids. However, even in the cold, aliphatic diazonium salts are unstable and easily breakdown into a variety of compounds.

$$NaNO_2 \ + \ HCl \longrightarrow HONO + \ NaCl$$

$$R\text{-}NH_2 \ + \ HONO \longrightarrow ROH + \ N_2 \ + \ H_2O$$
Primary amine   Alcohol

$$CH_3\text{-}NH_2 \ + \ HONO \longrightarrow CH_3OH + \ N_2 \ + \ H_2O$$
Methylamine   Methanol

(b) **Secondary amines** N-nitrosoamines are yellow, neutral oily chemicals that are insoluble in dilute aqueous mineral acids when they react with nitrous acid.

$$R_2NH \ + \ HONO \longrightarrow R\text{---}\underset{\underset{\displaystyle R}{|}}{N}\text{---}N\text{=}O \ + \ H_2O$$
Secondary amine   N-Nitrosoamine
                                      (yellow oil)

$$(CH_3)_2NH \ + \ HONO \longrightarrow H_3C\text{---}\underset{\underset{\displaystyle CH_3}{|}}{N}\text{---}N\text{=}O \ + \ H_2O$$
Dimethylamine   N-Nitrodimethylamine
                                      (yellow oil)

Nitrosomaines generate a green-colored solution when heated with a phenol crystal and a few drops of conc.H_2SO_4. When you dilute the solution, it turns red, but when you add a few drops of alkali, it turns deep blue.

(c) Water soluble amine salts are formed when tertiary aliphatic amines combine with nitrous acid. There is no discernible change in the appearance of the reacting materials.

$$R_3N \ + \ HONO \longrightarrow R_3\overset{+}{N}H\overset{-}{N}O_2$$
Tertiary amine   Trialkylammonium nitrite
                                      (soluble)

$$(CH_3)_3N \ + \ HONO \longrightarrow (CH_3)_3\overset{+}{N}H\overset{-}{N}O_2$$
Trimethylamine   Trimethylammonium nitrite
                                      (soluble)

3. **Hinsberg's method**: In the presence of sodium hydroxide, the amine mixture is treated with p-toluenesulphonyl chloride, also known as tosyl chloride (TSCl) or Hinsberg's reagent.

The **primary amines** react with mono-alkyl sulphonamide which dissolves in sodium hydroxide with the formation of sodium salt.

p-Toulene sulphonyl chloride

N-alkyl sulphonamide

Sod. salt of N-alkyl sulphonamide (Soluble)

Diakylsulphonamide is formed by the secondary amines and is insoluble in alkali.

p-Toulene sulphonyl chloride

N,N-dialkyl sulphonamide
(Insoluble in alkali)

The tertiary amines do not react at all.

On the basis of product obtained it is possible to distinguish between various classes of amines.

Preparation of amines:

Amines can be prepared by several methods which are discussed as follows:

1. **Reduction of nitriles:** Aliphatic primary amines can be made by catalytic hydrogenation or using chemical reducing agents to reduce nitriles.

$$R-C\equiv N \; + \; 3H_2 \xrightarrow[\text{heat}]{\text{Ni}} RCH_2NH_2$$

Nitrile

Primary amine

$$C_3H_7-C\equiv N \; + \; 3H_2 \xrightarrow[\text{heat}]{\text{Ni}} RCH_2NH_2$$

n-Butyronitrile

n-Butyl amine

2. Reduction of oximes and amides: Chemical or catalytic reduction of oximes and amides can also be used to make aliphatic amines.

$$RHC{=}NOH \quad + \quad 4H \xrightarrow{\text{Na, } C_2H_5OH} RCH_2NH_2 \quad + \quad H_2O$$

Aldoxmine   Primary amine

$$\underset{R}{\overset{R}{>}}C{=}NOH \quad + \quad 4H \xrightarrow{\text{Na, } C_2H_5OH} R{-}\overset{R}{\underset{}{C}}HNH_2 \quad + \quad H_2O$$

Ketoxime   Primary amine

$$R{-}\overset{O}{\overset{\|}{C}}{-}NH_2 \xrightarrow{\text{LiAlH}_4, H_3O^-} RCH_2NH_2$$

Amide   Primary amine

3. Gabriel Phthalimide reaction: Gabriel The phthalimide approach is a good way to make pure aliphatic or aralkyl primary amines. In this process, phthalimide is transformed to its potassium salt by treating it with alcoholic potassium hydroxide, which then forms N-substituted phthalimide when heated with an alkyl or aralkyl halide. Treatment with 20% HCl solution or refluxing with alkali solution hydrolyzes N-substituted phthalimide to give phthalic acid and a primary amine.

Phthalimide $\xrightarrow[{-H_2O}]{KOH}$ Potassium phthalimide $\xrightarrow[{-KX}]{RX}$ N-Alkylphthalimide $\rightarrow$ Phthalic acid + RNH$_2$ (Primary amine)

4. Hofmann Bromamide reaction: When amide is treated in an alkali solution with bromine or chlorine, it generates an amine with one less carbon atom than the initial amide.

$$R{-}\overset{O}{\overset{\|}{C}}{-}NH_2 \quad + \quad Br_2 \quad + \quad 4KOH \longrightarrow RNH_2 \quad + \quad K_2CO_3 \quad + \quad 2KBr \quad + 2H_2O$$

Amide   Amine

In this reaction, the hypobromite ion, OBr⁻, produced by an alkaline bromine solution (or the hypochlorite ion produced by an alkaline chlorine solution) initiates the reaction by attacking the amide, which is followed by the following steps:

$$Br_2 + 2KOH \longrightarrow KOBr + KBr + H_2O$$

1) $R-CONH_2 + OBr^- \longrightarrow R-CO-NH-Br + OH^-$

2) $R-CO-NH-Br + OH^- \longrightarrow R-CO-N^-Br + H_2O$

3) $R-CO-N^-Br \longrightarrow R-CO-N + Br^-$

4) $R-CO-N \longrightarrow R-N=C=O$

Step (1) involves the halogenation of amide to form an N-haloamide.

In step (2), hydroxide ion abstracts a hydrogen ion from N-haloamide.

In step (3), the anion formed undergoes elimination of bromide ion to form unstable species containing an electron deficient nitrogen known as nitrene

In step (4) nitrene undergoes 1,2-shift of alkyl group to nitrogen to yield an isocyanate.

In step (5) isocyanate undergoes hydrolysis to form amine and carbonate anion.

$$R-N=C=O + 2OH^- \longrightarrow R-NH_2 + CO_3^{2-}$$
isocyanate   amine   carbonate ion

5. **Reductive amination of aldehydes and ketones:** At a temperature of around 373K and 150 atm. pressure, aldehydes and ketones react with ammonia in the presence of a catalyst such as nickel.

$$R-CHO + NH_3 \xrightarrow{-H_2O} \left[R-CH=NH \right] \xrightarrow{H_2,Ni} RCH_2NH_2$$
Aldehyde   Aldimine   Primary amine

$$R-CO-R' + NH_3 \xrightarrow{-H_2O} \left[R-C(R')=NH \right] \xrightarrow{H_2,Ni} RR'CHNH_2$$
Ketone   Ketimine   Primary amine

6. **Ammonolysis of alcohols**: A mixture including primary, secondary, and tertiary amines is generated by heating an alcohol and ammonia combination in a sealed tube in the presence of copper chromite or alumina catalyst.

$$ROH + NH_3 \xrightarrow{\text{Alumina}} RNH_2 + H_2O$$

Alcohol · Primary amine

$$ROH + RNH_2 \longrightarrow R_2NH + H_2O$$

Secondary amine

$$ROH + R_2NH \longrightarrow R_3N + H_2O$$

Tertiary amine

7. **Curtius rearrangement**: The Curtius rearrangement is a reaction in which an acyl azide is generated by reacting an acyl halide with sodium azide (NaN_3) and then heated in an inert solvent. On heating, acyl azide loses a moelcule of nitrogen and becomes alkyl isocyanate, which, after further hydrolysis, yields primary amine.

$$R-\overset{O}{\overset{||}{C}}-Cl + NaN_3 \longrightarrow R-\overset{O}{\overset{||}{C}}-N_3$$

$$R-\overset{O}{\overset{||}{C}}-N_3 \xrightarrow[-N_2]{\text{Heat}} R-N=C=O \xrightarrow{H_2O} RNH_2 + CO_2$$

Alkyl isocyanate · Primary amine

Chemical Properties of Amines

1. **Basic nature**: Amines are bases because they have a lone pair of electrons on the nitrogen atom that are available for donation and protonation. Amines and acids combine to generate salts.

$$CH_3CH_2NH_2 + HCl \longrightarrow CH_3CH_2\overset{\oplus}{N}H_3\overset{-}{C}l$$

Ethylamine · Ethylammonium chloride

2. **Alkylation**: Amines are alkylated when they are exposed to alkyl halides. The initial amine transforms into higher-class amines, which then transform into quatenary ammonium halides.

   Exhaustive alkylation is the process of turning a given amine into a quaternary ammonium salt by reacting it with an alkyl halide.

$$RNH_2 \xrightarrow[-HX]{RX} R_2NH \xrightarrow[-HX]{RX} R_3N \xrightarrow[-HX]{RX} R_4\overset{+}{N}\overset{-}{X}$$

1^0 amine · 2^0 amine · 3^0 amine · Quaternary salts

3. **Conversion into amides**: Acylation: N-substituted amides are formed when primary and secondary amines react with acid chlorides or acid anhydrides. The acylation of amines is the process of converting amines to their amides.

Acetyl chloride + Methylamine → N-methylactamide

+ HCl

4. **Conversion into sulphonamides**: Primary and secondary amines react with sulphonyl chlorides such as benzenesulphonyl chloride and p-toluene sulphonyl chloride to form substituted sulphonamides.

p-Toulene sulphonyl chloride + H_2NR $\xrightarrow{-HCl}$ N-alkyl sulphonamide

NaOH

+ H_2O

Sod. salt of N-alkyl sulphonamide (Soluble)

p-Toulene sulphonyl chloride + NHR_2 → N,N-dialkyl sulphonamide (Insoluble in alkali) + HCl

5. **Reaction with nitrous acid**: The three classes of amines react with nitrous acid to produce three distinct compounds, as follows:

(a) Diaznoum salts are formed when primary aliphatic amines combine with cold nitrous acids. However, even in the cold, aliphatic diazonium salts are unstable and easily breakdown into a variety of compounds.

$$NaNO_2 + HCl \longrightarrow HONO + NaCl$$

$$R\text{-}NH_2 + HONO \longrightarrow ROH + N_2 + H_2O$$

Primary amine   Alcohol

$$CH_3\text{-}NH_2 + HONO \longrightarrow CH_3OH + N_2 + H_2O$$

Methylamine   Methanol

(b) Secondary amines react with nitrous acid to form N-nitrosoamines, which are oily, yellow molecules that are insoluble in dilute aqueous mineral acids.

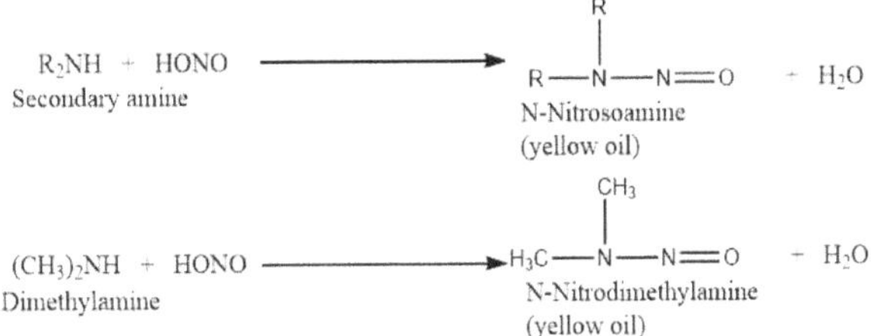

Nitrosomaines generate a green-colored solution when heated with a phenol crystal and a few drops of conc.H_2SO_4. When you dilute the solution, it turns red, but when you add a few drops of alkali, it turns deep blue.

(c) Water soluble amine salts are formed when tertiary aliphatic amines combine with nitrous acid. There is no discernible change in the appearance of the reacting materials.

$$R_3N \ + \ HONO \longrightarrow R_3\overset{+}{N}H\overset{-}{N}O_2$$

Tertiary amine

Trialkylammonium nitrite (soluble)

$$(CH_3)_3N \ + \ HONO \longrightarrow (CH_3)_3\overset{+}{N}H\overset{-}{N}O_2$$

Trimethylamine

Trimethylammonium nitrite (soluble)

6. Carbylamine reaction:

When primary amine interacts with chloroform and alcoholic potash, it forms an alkyl isocyanide (or carbylamine), which has a strong odour.

$$R\text{-}NH_2 \ + \ CHCl_3 + \ 3KOH \longrightarrow R\text{—}\overset{+}{N}\equiv\overset{-}{C} \ + \ 3KCl \ + \ 3H_2O$$

1^0 amine

Isocyanate

7. Action of carbon disulphide:

When amines are warmed with carbon disulphide in the presence of mercuric chloride, aliphatic primary amines yield isothiocyanate which smells like mustard oil.

$$R\text{—}NH_2 \ + \ CS_2 \xrightarrow{\text{heat}} RHN\text{—}\overset{\overset{\displaystyle S}{\|}}{C}\text{—}SH \longrightarrow RNCS \ + \ HgS \ + \ HCl$$

Primary amine

Dithiocarbamic acid

Alkyl isocyanate

Some important amines with its uses:

Ethanolamine

Chemical formula: C_2H_7NO

Uses:

1. Detergents, emulsifiers, polishes, medicines, corrosion inhibitors, and chemical intermediates are all made from it.

2. It is used in cosmetics as a pH regulator.

3. Ethanolamine is commonly used to alkalinize water in power plants' steam cycles, particularly nuclear reactors with pressurised water reactors.

4. Ethanolamine is largely utilised in pharmaceutical formulations for buffering and emulsion preparation.

5. Ethanolamines are used in personal care goods and cosmetics as washing agents, or surfactants. Ethanolamines assist eliminate dirt and oil from the skin by dissolving grease and combining other vital chemicals in these types of lotions.

6. It can be employed in industrial settings like chemical production and gas treatment. It aids in the removal of pollutants from gasoline in gas treatment operations for refineries and natural gas streams.

Ethylenediamine:

Chemical formula: $C_2H_8N_2$

1. Ethylenediamine is a major derivative of ethylenediamine, which is used to make the chelating agent EDTA.

2. Ethylenediamine is a component of the bronchodilator aminophylline, where it helps to dissolve the active ingredient theophylline. In dermatological preparations, ethylenediamine has also been employed.

3. It's been utilised as a urinary acidifier in the past.

4. Ethylenediamine is a chemical that is used to make first-generation antihistamines (piperoxan).

5. Ethylenediamine is a widely utilised polymer precursor since it has two amine groups. Plasticizers are formaldehyde-derived condensates. It's a common ingredient in polyurethane fibre manufacture.

6. It's also utilised in paints and coolants as a corrosion inhibitor.

Amphetamine

Chemical formula: $C_9H_{13}N$

Attention deficit hyperactivity disorder (ADHD), narcolepsy, and obesity are all treated with amphetamine (alpha-methylphenethylamine), a powerful central nervous system stimulant.

Uses:

1. Amphetamine is used to treat ADHD, narcolepsy (sleep disorder), and obesity.

2. Amphetamine is utilised by some athletes to improve their psychological and athletic performance, such as endurance and attentiveness.

3. At therapeutic levels, amphetamine produces emotional and cognitive effects like exhilaration and a shift in sexual desire.

4. It can cause exhilaration and inhibit the appetite, resulting in weight reduction.

5. Amphetamine has been used to treat a wide range of ailments. It is now mostly used to treat ADHD and, in rare occasions, depression.

6. Amphetamine is a medication that is used recreationally. It is used to promote libido, wakefulness, cognitive control, sociability, and generate euphoria in people. It can also improve reaction times, muscle strength, and tiredness reduction.

MCQs

1. The correct order of decreasing acid strength of trichloroacetic acid (A), trifluoro acetic acid (B), acetic acid (C) and formic acid.

   (a) $A > B > C > D$

   (b) $A > C > B > D$

   (c) $B > A > D > C$

   (d) $B > D > C > A$

2. The Hinsberg's method is used for which of the following

   (a) Preparation of primary amine

   (b) Preparation of secondary amines

   (c) Preparation of tertiary amines

   (d) Separation of amine mixture

3. Acetic acid is obtained when which of the given reaction take place?

   (a) Methyl alcohol is oxidized with potassium permanganate

   (b) Calcium acetate is distilled in the presence of calcium formate

   (c) Acetaldehyde is oxidized with potassium dichromate and sulphuric acid

   (d) Glycerol is heated with sulphuric acid

4. Acetamide is treated separately with the following reagents. Which one of these would give methylamines?

   (a) PCl_5

   (b) $NaOH + Br_2$

   (c) Sodalime

   (d) Hot Conc. H_2SO_4

5. Correct structure of Amphetamine

6. Correct structure of Lactic acid.

   a) 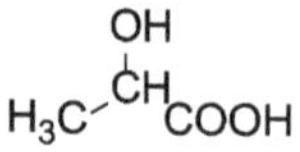 $H_3C-\overset{\overset{\displaystyle OH}{|}}{CH}-COOH$

   b) 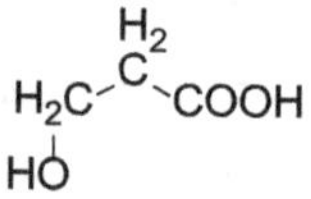 $H_2C-\overset{H_2}{\underset{\underset{\displaystyle HO}{|}}{C}}-COOH$

   c) $H_2C\overset{\displaystyle OH}{\diagup}$, $H_3C-\overset{\overset{\displaystyle}{|}}{CH}-COOH$

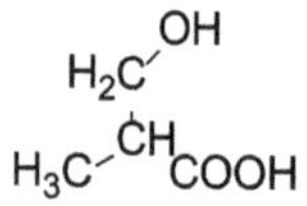

   d) 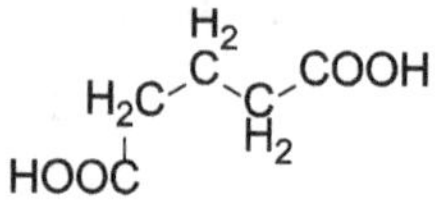 $H_2C-\overset{H_2}{C}-\overset{COOH}{\underset{\underset{\displaystyle HOOC}{|}}{C}H_2}$

7. Which compound has the highest boiling point?

   (a) CH_3CH_3

   (b) CH_3OCH_3

   (c) CH_3CH_2OH

   (d) CH_3COOH

8. The greater acidity of carboxylic acids compared to alcohols arises primarily from:-

   (a) The electron-donating effect of hydroxyl group

   (b) The electron-withdrawing effect of the carbonyl oxygen

   (c) The acidity of α-hydrogens of carboxylic acids

   (d) The resonance stability associated with the carboxylate ion

9. Which of the following is the strongest acid?

   (a) Formic acid

   (b) Trichloroacetic acid

   (c) Acetic acid

   (d) Trifluoroacetic acid

10. Which of the following is the strongest acid?

   (a) Butanoic acid

   (b) 2-Chlorobutanoic acid

   (c) 3-Chlorobutanoic acid

   (d) 4-Chlorobutanoic acid

11. Correct structure of acetic acid:

   (a) CH_3CH_2CHO

   (b) CH_3COOH

   (c) CH_3CH_2COOH

   (d) $CH_3CH_2CH_2COOH$

12. Correct structure of succinic acid is:

   a) 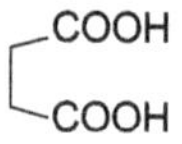 (structure with two COOH groups)

   b) 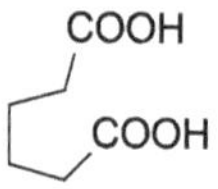 (structure with two COOH groups)

   c) 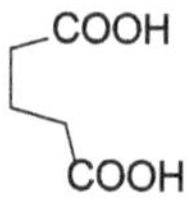 (structure with two COOH groups)

   d) 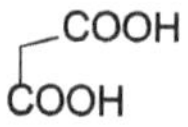 (structure with two COOH groups)

13. Lowest value of pKa:

    (a) Acetic acid   (b) 2-chlorobutanoic acid

    (c) 2-chlorobutanoic acid   (d) Trichloroacetic acid

14. Correct structure for Ethylenediamine

    (a) $NH_2CH_2NH_2$ (b) $CH_3NHNHCH_3$

    (c) $NH_2CH_2CH_2NH_2$ (d) None of the above

15. Correct structure of benzoic acid.

a) benzene ring with COOH

b) benzene ring with COOH and CH_3

c) benzene ring with COOH and CHO

d) benzene ring with COOH and OCH_3

16. Which among the following is a not derivative of carboxylic acids.

    (a) Ester   (b) Amide

    (c) Aldehyde   (d) Anhydride

17. The products of the reaction:

phthalimide (NK) $\xrightarrow[H_2O]{RX}$?

    (a) RNH_2 (b) R_2NH

    (c) R_3Ns (d) All of these.

Answers for MCQs

1. (a)	2. (d)	3. (c)	4. (b)	5. (b)
6. (a)	7. (d)	8. (d)	9. (d)	10. (b)
11. (b)	12. (a)	13. (d)	14. (c)	15. (a)
16. (c)	17. (a)			

Short Answer Questions

1. What are carboxylic acids? Write the formulae of the two simplest aliphatic carboxylic acids and give their IUPAC names.

2. Arrange the following acids in increasing order of acidic character:

   Pentanoic acid, 2-bromopentanoic acid and 3-bromopentanoic acid.

3. Compare the acidic character of o-chlorobenzoic acid and p-chlorobenzoic acid.

4. Account for the fact that C-O bond length is shorter in RCOOH than in ROH.

5. Explain why most of carboxylic acids exist as cyclic dimers.

6. Benzoic acid reacts with sodium bicarbonate to give CO_2 but phenols donot. Justify your answer.

7. Which out of benzoic acid and formic acid is a stronger acid. Explain.

8. How will you prepare the following:

   (i)   Benzoic acid from benzene

   (ii) Benzoyl chloride from benzoic acid.

9. Explain why trichloroacetic acid stronger acid than acetic acid.

10. Write down the qualitative test used for the identification of carboxylic acids.

11. Write down the reactions for the conversion of carboxylic acids into amides, esters, acid chlorides and acid anhydrides.

12. Why are carboxylic acids stronger acids as compared to phenols?

13. What is Hunsdiecker reaction?

14. Why is ammonia less basic than aromatic amines?

15. Explain why aniline is weaker base than methylamine.

16. How can you distinguish between aniline and acetamide.

17. What is Hinsberg's reagent?

Long Answer Questions

1. Discuss the effect of substituents on the acidity of aliphatic carboxylic acids.

2. Write short notes on the following:

   (i)   Hunsdiecker reaction

   (ii) Decarboxylation of carboxylic acids.

3. Write down any five preparations of carboxylic acids.

4. Discuss chemical reactions of carboxylic acids showing the acidic character of carboxylic acids.

5. What are amines? How are they named and classified?

6. Write down methods to separate various classes of amines.

7. Discuss the factors effecting basicity of amines. Also explain why basicity order is as a result of solvation effect and inductive effect.

8. Explain along with reactions various qualitative test for esters.

9. Briefly discuss Gabriel Phthalimide synthesis reaction.

10. Write a short note on Hofmann degradation of amides.

11. What are primary, secondary and tertiary amines? How are these distinguished from each other?

12. Write down atleast four methods used for the preparation of amines.

13. Discuss important chemical reactions of amines.

14. Arrange the following in decreasing order of boiling points:

    Primary, secondary, tertiary amines with same number of carbon atoms.

References

[1] Morrison RT, Boyd RN. Organic Chemistry, 6th ed., Pearson Education Inc., New Jersey; 2002, ISBN-81-203-0765-8.

[2] Bahl A, Bahl BS. Advanced Organic Chemistry, S. Chand and Company Limited, India; 2010, ISBN: 8121935156, 9788121935159.

[3] Klein DR. Organic Chemistry, 3rd ed., John Wiley and Sons Inc., United States of America, 2017; ISBN 978-1-119-31615-2.

[4] Carey FA, Giuliano RM, Allison NT, Bane SL. Organic Chemistry, 11th ed., McGraw-Hill Education, New York, 2019, ISBN: 1260565874, 9781260565874.

[5] Rawn, JD, Ouellette RJ. Organic Chemistry: Structure, Mechanism and Synthesis, 2nd ed., Academic Press, United Kingdon, 2018, ISBN: 0128128380, 9780128128381.

[6] Smith JG. Organic Chemistry, 6th ed., McGraw-Hill Education, New York, 2018, ISBN: 1260119106, 9781260119107.

[7] Clayden J, Greeves N, Warren SG. Organic Chemistry, 2nd ed., Oxford University Press, New York, 2012, ISBN 978-0-19-927029-3.

[8] McMurry JE. Organic Chemistry, ninth ed., Cengage Learning, United States of America, 2015, ISBN: 1305080483, 9781305080485.

[9] Solomons TWG, Fryhle SA. Snyder, Organic Chemistry, 11th ed., Wiley, United States of America, 2013, ISBN 978-1-118-13357-6.

[10] Brown WH, Iverson BL, Anslyn E, Foote CS. Organic Chemistry, 8th ed., Brooks Cole, United States, 2017, ISBN: 1305580354, 9781305580350.

[11] Bruice PY. Organic Chemistry, eight ed., Pearson Education, Santa Barbara, 2017, ISBN: 9780134042282.

[12] https://www.researchgate.net/publication/229973499_The_Perkin_Reaction_and_Related _Reactions (accessed 22 October 2020).

[13] https://shodhganga.inflibnet.ac.in/bitstream/10603/154947/12/12_chapter%203.pdf (accessed 22 October 2020).

[14] Vollhardt KPC, Schore NE. Organic Chemistry: Structure and Function, 8th ed., W. H. Freeman, New York, 2018, ISBN: 1319188966, 9781319188962.

[15] Kar A. Advanced Organic Chemistry: Structure and Mechanism, 1st ed., MedTech, India, 2017, ISBN: 9789387025202.

[16] Lewis DE. Advanced Organic Chemistry, Oxford University Press, New York, 2016, ISBN: 9780199758975, 0199758972.